SPECIAL DIET COOKBOOKS

CANDIDA ALBICANS

D0170056

SPECIAL DIET COOKBOOKS

CANDIDA ALBICANS

Yeast-free recipes for renewed health and vitality

Richard Turner and Elizabeth Simonsen

THORSONS PUBLISHING GROUP

First published 1987 by Viking O'Neil, Penguin Books Australia Ltd
This revised UK edition first published 1989

British Library Cataloguing in Publication Data

Turner, Richard
Candida albicans: yeast free recipes for
renewed health and vitality. — (Special
diet cookbooks)
1. Food. Yeast-free dishes. Recipes
I. Title.   II. Simonsen, Elizabeth.
III. Series
641.5'632

ISBN 0-7225-1718-1

Published by Thorsons Publishers Limited,
Wellingborough, Northamptonshire, NN8 2RQ, England.

Printed and bound in Great Britain by
Mackays of Chatham PLC, Chatham, Kent

3 5 7 9 8 6 4

Contents

A Note From the Authors

It has concerned me for many years that, as a pharmacist, I have been called upon to dispense prescriptions to patients knowing that the medication prescribed may cause side-effects more unpleasant than the condition being treated. I was further concerned by the attitude of many, that all ailments could be cured by simply 'popping' the appropriate pill. My concern led me to believe that there had to be a better way.

Studying for my Diploma of Orthomolecular Nutrition introduced me to an awareness of the importance of nutrition and diet in health and disease and to the concept of prevention of disease by diet and lifestyle modification. Further research in this area of study revealed Candidiasis as a potentially serious medical problem whose incidence was growing rapidly and which responded dramatically to diet and lifestyle modification. The frustration caused by the lack of a simply-understood explanation of the condition and a positive diet guide prompted me to do something about it. This book is the result.

Richard Turner
B.Pharm. M.P.S.

In the late 1970s, I was working as a dietitian in a practice where 60 per cent of the patients were overweight and on traditional weight-reduction diets. There were a few people who, try as they might, were unable to lose weight on a regular 1200 kilojoule* diet. This puzzled me. In searching for a solution to the problem I suggested a diet free of yeast-containing products. To my surprise, in many cases, it worked dramatically, and with some interesting side effects.

Women who had 'thrush' reported relief from their symptoms. Others who had been suffering abdominal discomfort, pre-menstrual tension, and hot flushes also found that they were no longer bothered with these problems. Could this be just coincidence? I explained the yeast-free diet to other patients and many were willing to try it. Yes, they reported similar results: disappearance of headaches, relief from indigestion or from that ache or pain they had learned to live with.

I discussed this with colleagues who found it quite unusual, but then I found that similar work was being done in the United States and in Britain. I soon discovered that there were many people who felt chronically unwell, but who medical tests indicated were quite healthy. In a large number of cases a yeast-free diet was putting them back on the road to good health. From my own experience and research, along with work being done by people around the world, this book has emerged.

Elizabeth Simonsen
Registered Dietitian

* 1 kilojoule = approx. 0.25 calorie.

Introduction

This book is about yeasts and the detrimental effect they can have on human health. *Candida albicans* is a usually harmless yeast organism which lives on the skin and mucous membranes of the body. It has long been recognised as the cause of 'thrush'. However, there is growing evidence in the USA, Britain and Australia that yeasts, such as Candida, may be responsible for a wide range of medical disorders and that the incidence of yeast-related illness is increasing.

When the delicate balance of yeasts and bacteria within the human ecosystem is disturbed, the debilitating disease, chronic Candidiasis can occur. Many factors can produce such an imbalance. In the past thirty to forty years, yeast-related illnesses have become more common. Why? It appears that changes in lifestyle, medicine and diet during this century have all been major contributors.

There is much to be grateful for in modern medicine; many scourges of the past have disappeared and many painful and often fatal illnesses can now be relieved or cured. However, in some cases, ridding the body of Problem A has caused Problem B to arise. Long term treatment with antibiotics can produce a yeast imbalance. While destroying the bacteria in the body which was causing disease, antibiotics may also destroy the naturally occurring bacteria whose job is to keep yeasts in balance. Also, it is now clear that long term use of the contraceptive pill can produce an overgrowth or 'flare up' of organisms such as *Candida albicans*. The pill was unheard of thirty years ago: now it is commonplace.

The combined effect of these two factors can produce a yeast imbalance so great that it is impossible for a normal immune system to eradicate, and can produce a sufficient quantity of toxins to chronically poison the host individual. Clearly, a more thoughtful and cautious approach to modern technology and lifestyle is needed by some people.

The regular consumption of what used to be regarded as special foods has also contributed to the recent increase in yeast-related health problems. Until midway through this century, high carbohydrate foods were made for celebrations: birthdays, weddings, religious holidays. Today, it is possible to have cakes, different breads and sweets every day. They can be picked up at the corner store or supermarket. Yeasts thrive on simple carbohydrates and, where an imbalance exists, such foods will contribute further to the problem.

Candida is opportunistic. It exacerbates existing illnesses and invades where there is a weakness. Thus, where an imbalance occurs, the toxins from yeast may produce increasing pain in the joints where a previous injury occurred, worsening arthritis, headaches, digestive upsets. Yeast toxins have no specific target, but can poison virtually any cell or organ in the body. Consequently, they can produce an extremely wide range of symptoms in people of either sex and of any age. However, some symptoms tend to point more directly to Candidiasis.

If you, or a member of your family have been putting up with any one or more of the following symptoms, you may be a victim of the insidious Candida: recurrent or persistent infections of the vagina or urinary tract, period pain, irregular menstrual bleeding, depression, pre-menstrual syndrome, explosive temper outbursts or hyperactivity, sleeplessness, persistent rashes or infections of the skin, weight gain or loss, food cravings, heartburn, diarrhoea, constipation or other digestive problems, or breathing problems aggravated by pollution or damp, humid weather.

This book will provide you with information on the causes, diagnosis and treatment of Candida infection and infestation. A clear plan for combatting the effects of yeast imbalance is outlined, based on a yeast-free, low carbohydrate diet. If, after consultation, you adopt the anti-Candida regime, you will find that the diet, in combination with the other treatments suggested, will put you on the road to renewed health and vigour.

It is absolutely vital that you first consult your doctor and have a thorough medical examination to rule out the possibility of other causes for any of the symptoms mentioned. If, however, you find there is no identifiable reason for the fact that you simply feel unwell, then the *Candida Albicans* special diet cookbook may provide the answer.

CHAPTER 1

Profile on *Candida albicans*

Over 2,000 years ago, Hippocrates, the father of modern medicine, described in his writings, a condition of the mouth and the vagina known as 'thrush'. It was not until the 1850s, after Louis Pasteur developed the germ theory of disease, that the cause of this condition was identified as an infection of the skin or of the lining of the vagina or mouth by a microscopic organism known as *Candida albicans* (sometimes known as *Monilia albicans*).

Candida albicans, is a microscopic, single-celled organism. It is a member of a sub-group of yeasts belonging to the family of fungi or moulds. You will be quite familiar with fungi as mushrooms and as the 'fur' which grows on spoiling bread or fruit. Yeasts too are familiar. They have been used for thousands of years to process various foods. Baker's yeast is the ingredient which is necessary to make dough rise prior to the baking of bread. The yeast is mixed with flour and water and left in a warm place for a time while the enzymes released by the yeast 'digest' or ferment the starch and produce thousands of tiny bubbles of carbon dioxide gas. This in turn, causes the dough to rise and gives the bread its light, aerated consistency. In the liquor industry, brewer's yeast is mixed with crushed grapes in a vat and allowed to ferment the grape sugar to produce alcohol and carbon dioxide gas. The gas may be trapped in the case of champagne, or allowed to escape to produce a still wine. In both instances, the yeast releases enzymes which ferment carbohydrates.

Moulds have their place in the biological world, acting as the carrion of their microscopic environment where their enzymes contribute to the continual rotting and breakdown of dead organisms and the regeneration of the supply of nutrients to living organisms. These microscopic organisms, in large numbers, constitute a complex chemical powerhouse with the potential to manufacture huge quantities of some chemicals such as alcohol, and minute quantities of thousands of other chemicals, many of which are unique to one particular yeast or mould species.

Yeasts are very widespread in our environment, occurring naturally in the soil and on the surfaces of almost all living organisms. They are part of the delicate microscopic ecosystem of minute living beings which exist in a sort of love-hate relationship with each other. Each one tolerates the other as long as the ecosystem remains in balance and no one part of the system becomes dominant over any other part.

Each one of us has, living on our skin surfaces, a blend of yeast and other micro-organisms which live in harmony with each other and with their host. The linings of the human body (mucous membranes) are extensions of the external skin and can also host a cocktail of various micro-organisms without causing the least discomfort or disease. *Candida albicans* has been isolated from the skin and from the mucous membrane linings of the digestive tract and upper respiratory tract and vagina without causing any untoward reactions. However, as with any ecosystem, when the natural balance is disturbed by the introduction of an external influence, the resulting effects may be more widespread than anticipated.

Candida albicans occurs as spores and in two actively growing forms. It occurs in the more normal form where it reproduces by the yeast cell budding new cells, or it can occur as a filimentous or 'mycelial' form. When a disturbance of the normal level of Candida on our skin or mucous membranes occurs, a range of common symptoms appears: the discharge and itching of vulvo-vaginitis (vaginal thrush), the white coated tongue of oral thrush, oesophagitis (heartburn) and the abdominal discomfort, distension, constipation, diarrhoea and rectal itching that goes with yeast infection of the bowel.

Dr Orian Truss, a pioneer in research into yeast-related illness, observed that, in many of his patients for whom he successfully treated Candida infections, several other seemingly unrelated, often vague symptoms co-incidentally disappeared when the Candida infection cleared. In his book *The Missing Diagnosis*, he reported his observations and suggested that the widespread use of antibiotics, combined with the use of birth control pills and of immunosuppressant (cortisone type) medication, coupled with a prolonged high, simple carbohydrate diet (fast food type) has caused a dramatic change in that delicate relationship between Candida and the other micro-organisms which co-exist on our skin and mucous membranes. All of these factors tend to suppress the organisms which compete with Candida, discourage the body's own immune system to correct the imbalance, or encourage Candida to flourish. This causes such a disturbance to the fragile ecosystem as to be a major cause of the disease which is outwardly benign, yet can be so debilitating; that of chronic Candidiasis.

CHAPTER 2
Candida and the Immune System

Allergies or intolerances to substances in our environment are not a new phenomenon. Again, Hippocrates observed over 2,000 years ago that the consumption of certain foods resulted in a severe reaction in some people. However, it would appear that in recent times, there has been an accelerating frequency and severity of such reactions to foods and environmental chemicals.

Under normal circumstances, our body's immune system will be activated when the body is invaded by any matter which it can identify as being foreign. The foreign matter may be pollen, bacteria, moulds, viruses, chemical pollutants in the air, chemicals applied to the skin, chemicals ingested with food, synthetic or natural, or even improperly digested food fragments. Whenever the body is invaded by foreign matter, a normal, competent immune system will isolate and destroy it and so protect all the other cells of the body from exposure to that potentially toxic matter. If, for any reason, the immune system fails to completely detoxify all foreign material entering the body, then that material is circulated throughout the body by the bloodstream. It can then bring about an aberration in the biochemistry of various body cells which may be expressed as unpleasant symptoms such as congestion of the sinuses, precipitation of an asthma attack, alteration of mood or behaviour, headache, or a whole host of other symptoms. As the toxins affect the functioning of individual cells, there is a tendency for the symptoms not to be confined to one particular body system, such as the circulatory system, but to be more general in nature. There is, however, a tendency for symptoms to be focused on an individual's weaknesses, so that if there is a familial history of arthritis or asthma then these are the groups of cells in which the toxins are most likely to cause aberration of their biochemistry and thus likely to produce symptoms.

The ability of each individual's body to cope with or succumb to the toxic effects of foreign material is solely dependent on the ability of one's immune system to cope with that foreign material and is influenced by many factors.

1 **Adequate nutrition.** Like all body systems, the immune system, to function efficiently, must have an adequate supply of the whole range of nutrients, particularly vitamins A, B6 and C and zinc in the correct proportions. A well balanced diet will supply these nutrients.

2 **Stress.** Whenever the body is exposed to any form of stress, whether it is physical stress caused by infection or injury, or emotional stress, chemical changes occur in the body which have a suppressant effect upon the immune system.

3 **Allergenic load.** One's allergenic load is the total quantity of foreign material which has been permitted to invade the body. It is an expression of the workload that the immune system has to deal with. Substances which contribute to the allergenic load may be absorbed into the body in various ways. These include chemical pollutants inhaled with the air we breathe; dust, pollen, bacteria or mould spores inhaled; chemicals, either as pollutants or additives to the food we consume; and naturally occurring contaminants of food such as natural poisons, bacteria, yeasts and viruses or products of their breakdown. Many chemical pollutants increase the incidence of abnormal cells within the body and it is the responsibility of the immune system to identify and destroy these.

Like all living beings, the yeast cell is extremely complex. Thousands of chemical reactions are going on inside each cell all the time and each reaction is an integral part of the life process of that cell. As with all living beings, many of these chemicals (metabolites) are wastes and are expelled. When the yeast is living in the gut, metabolites are released and may be absorbed into the bloodstream and circulated throughout the body. When the yeast dies and/or is digested another host of chemicals is released into the gut from which they may be absorbed into the bloodstream. Many of these chemicals have been positively identified as being toxic to the brain and capable of causing behavioural disturbances.

A particularly large amount of yeast metabolites can be provided by a diet which is high in yeast-based foods such as bread, cheese, beer or wine. The other major source of yeast metabolites is from a mass of *Candida albicans* living in the gut, unfettered by competing bacteria, and nourished by a diet which has a high proportion of simple carbohydrates. The quantity of metabolites obtained from these sources, either separately or combined, can become quite large, too large even for a healthy immune system to detoxify, much less an immune system which is in any way compromised by other factors such as food allergens or by immunosuppressant type medication. The problem can be further compounded by the introduction of yeast metabolites from other minor sources such as by the inhalation of moulds or mould spores (the musty smell in mouldy environments). These are trapped by the normal air cleansing mechanisms in the nasal and chest passages where they break down releasing yet more metabolites.

In a healthy gut, these chemicals would not be absorbed through the gut wall as it normally provides a sieve-type effect which allows only simple chemicals with small molecules to pass. However, in a gut which is infested with *Candida albicans* which changes to its mycelial form and burrows into the intestinal wall, the infestation may irritate the gut lining so much that it will lose its ability to act as an effective sieve and allows to pass through to the bloodstream many of the more complex chemicals. These are larger molecules and more likely to be foreign to the host and so contribute to the allergenic load.

A poor diet, high in refined, simple carbohydrates can compromise the immune system. It provides an inadequate supply of vitamins and minerals to sustain and nourish the system and encourages a 'flare up' or multiplication of *Candida albicans*.

CHAPTER 3

Diagnosis of Candida Imbalance

It is extremely important to realise that any of the symptoms described here can be the manifestation of many disorders other than those related to *Candida albicans* and it is imperative to have a thorough examination by your physician to rule out that possibility before making the assumption that the cause of your particular condition is Candida imbalance.

As Candida is present in almost everyone, healthy or ill, it is practically impossible to devise a laboratory test which will positively identify it as the causative agent of an illness. Some rather expensive blood tests can point to the possibility only that Candida is the cause of a specific condition. Diagnosis relies on the presence of symptoms, combined with the occurence of certain risk factors which only a thorough medical history would bring to light. Following the history taking, an accurate diagnosis can only be confirmed by an improvement in the condition as a result of instituting anti-Candida treatment. A diagnosis of chronic Candidiasis is likely to be made if a history reveals any of the following circumstances.

1 Repeated or prolonged courses of *broad spectrum antibiotics*, especially for repeated or recurrent sinus or ear infections, bronchitis or acne.
Broad spectrum antibiotics suppress those micro-organisms in the gut which live in competition with yeasts and thus allow the yeast colonies to flare up.

2 Courses of *Cortisone, Prednisolone* or other *Corticosteroids* for skin rashes, asthma or arthritis.
   These medications directly suppress the body's own natural immune system in its ability to prevent 'flare up' of yeasts anywhere in the body and in its ability to detoxify foreign matter such as food allergens or yeast metabolites.

3 *Multiple pregnancies*, the use of *birth control pills* or other *hormone preparations*.
   These produce a particular imbalance of hormones in the body which encourages yeast growth.

4 A prolonged *high carbohydrate diet*, especially of simple carbohydrates such as sugars and white flour preparations. Simple carbohydrates like these are the foods on which yeast cells thrive and therefore encourage a proliferation of yeast cells in the intestine.

In the experience of Candida infection sufferers all symptoms imaginable have been presented and have been relieved by anti-Candida treatment. However, some symptoms seem to appear more frequently in Candida patients' medical histories and these tend to pinpoint *Candida albicans* as the prime suspect.

1 Recurrent or chronic infections of the vagina or urinary system.
   These suggest a chronic Candida infection which often leads to other disorders of the urinary and sex organs such as fluid retention, endometriosis, period pain and cramps, irregular menstrual bleeding and an impairment or loss of sex drive.

2 Recurrent or chronic infections of the skin, especially around the finger and toe nails; recurrent 'athlete's foot' infection; 'jock itch' or psoriasis.

3 Depression in either sex, but especially in women, associated with a continual feeling of tiredness.
   This suggests a tired immune system. This may be associated with other vague nervous system symptoms such as inability

to concentrate, poor memory, headache, pre-menstrual tension, explosive temper outbursts, lack of co-ordination, irritability, drowsiness, loss of self confidence, crying spells, loss of reasoning ability or inability to sleep.

4 Cravings for sweet and carbohydrate rich foods which provide a supply of nutrients for the yeast colonies in the intestine: cravings for yeast-derived foods such as cheese, bread, yeast and malt extracts, and especially alcoholic beverages.
It is a common occurrence in allergy situations that the individual develops a craving or addiction to the actual item to which they are allergic.

5 Symptoms which are aggravated by tobacco smoke, car or diesel exhaust fumes, perfumes or other chemical odours.
In a healthy individual, these compounds are detoxified by the immune system before they produce any detectable results but in anyone with a compromised immune system they are free to cause damage at a cellular level and so produce symptoms.

6 Symptoms which are worse on damp, humid days or while in damp, mouldy environments.
At these times, the mould level in the atmosphere is much higher and there are far more mould spores floating about, being inhaled, broken down and absorbed, thus contributing to the allergenic load.

7 Persistent digestive problems.
This is the most common symptom of Candida-related problems in men. Heartburn, indigestion, bloating and gas, abdominal distension and pain, constipation or diarrhoea or alternating bouts of both are all symptoms which suggest a 'flare up' of yeast colonisation of the gastro-intestinal tract.

8 Recurrent sore throats, nasal congestion or cough.
These point to Candida colonisation of the sinuses.

Patients suffering post-viral syndrome or myalgic encephalo-myelitis have found an improvement in their condition when an anti-Candida program has been instituted as part of their therapy, suggesting that yeast must in some way contribute to their misery. Other vague symptoms which have been reported include pain and swelling in the joints, pain or tightness in the chest, blurred vision or spots before the eyes, ringing in the ears, cold extremities, or just plain 'feeling poorly' and have been reduced or have disappeared following anti-Candida treatment.

CHAPTER 4
How to Beat Candida

Candida can be very deceitful. The disease slowly creeps up on the unsuspecting patient, and then lies hidden under a cloak of confusingly vague symptoms and feelings. It gives a glimpse of itself here and there, but refuses to allow a simple diagnosis of the insidious condition it causes. Typically, Candida will not be wiped out by a simple course of antibiotics. It quickly re-establishes itself, simply because the immune system is too exhausted to cope with a 'flare up' of yeasts.

It is necessary to attempt to reverse all of the factors which led to the development of the Candida problem, to relieve the pressure on the immune system and allow it to recover from the constant bombardment by yeast metabolites and other toxic compounds including allergens and external poisons. Successful anti-Candida treatment attacks the problem in two ways. It reduces and suppresses the yeasts living in the gut and it allows the immune system to rest and recuperate. The basis of such treatment is the yeast-free, low carbohydrate diet outlined in detail in this book. Ideally, an overall approach to the Candida problem is the most effective and brings about improvement in the shortest time. Instituting part of the program will bring about improvement in some individuals who are less seriously affected. A holistic approach is recommended in the attempt to control the Candida infection and allow re-establishment of a competent immune system. As many as possible of the following treatment measures should be instituted.

1 Suppress the Yeast Living in the Gut

- Modify the diet and lifestyle to starve the offending yeast and thereby suppress its proliferation in the gut.
- Avoid medications which promote yeast growth such as the contraceptive pill, antibiotics and cortisone type medications.
- Take a specific anti-yeast antibiotic to rid the gut of the mass of Candida living there.

2 Rest and Stimulate the Immune System

- Avoid foods which are yeast derived and thus contain yeast metabolites.
- Identify and avoid chemicals and other foods to which you may be allergic.
- Avoid exposure to yeast spores in the atmosphere.
- Avoid medications which suppress the immune system such as cortisone and other immunosuppressant drugs.
- Use injections of extracts of *Candida albicans* to stimulate the immune system.
- Use vitamin and mineral supplements to nourish the immune system and assist its regeneration.
- Exercise.
- Think positively.

Starvation of Candida by Diet Modification

Yeasts thrive on highly processed carbohydrates such as simple sugars and starches. They can similarly be starved by denying them sugars and white flour products in the diet and by placing more emphasis on foods which are unprocessed and so have a higher percentage of complex carbohydrates. A yeast-free, low carbohydrate diet is fundamental to the anti-Candida program. Without diet modification, successful treatment is simply not possible. The greater part of this book is thus devoted to such a diet, which should be adopted in combination with all or any of the other treatment measures.

Avoidance of Yeast Promoting Medications

'Flare up' of Candida infection is actually encouraged by some prescribed medications which, if avoided, can significantly reduce yeast growth. Antibiotics, especially broad spectrum antibiotics, upset the normal bacteria-yeast ecosystem balance in the gut by suppressing the bacteria and allowing the yeasts to proliferate. Broad spectrum antibiotics are often used long-term for several chronic problems which may be manifestations· of allergy related disorders such as chronic acne, sinus infections or bronchial infections. The use of broad spectrum antibiotics allows the Candida in the gut to proliferate, placing a further load on an immune system already struggling to cope with the allergy causing agent.

Certain hormone preparations including the contraceptive pill and medication to relieve menopausal symptoms, alter the metabolic pattern in the body in a way which encourages yeast proliferation. Sometimes the problem is compounded when the oral contraceptive is combined with broad spectrum antibiotics to treat a chronic acne problem. It might also be noted that many of the menopausal symptoms treated by hormones are the same as those which have been associated with Candida.

The immunosuppressant and cortisone-type medications, as the name suggests, suppress the immune system. This renders it less able to cope with a chronic Candida infection. The cortisone-type drugs, usually prednisolone, prednisone and betamethasone are used to relieve immune system disorders which may be manifestations of an underlying Candida imbalance.

A single course of any of these medications can encourage a temporary 'flare up' of Candida infection without causing any untoward effects. However, these medications, being for chronic conditions, are often taken for years at a time and are sometimes taken in combination. All encourage yeast growth and therefore should be avoided when following this regime.

Suppression of Candida with a Specific Anti-yeast Antibiotic

The most commonly used specific anti-yeast antibiotic is nystatin (Mycostatin or Nilstat), which is a highly purified metabolite of the bacterium Streptomyces noursei. Nystatin is a bitter tasting pale yellow powder which is insoluble in water. It is available on prescription as capsules, tablets and in liquid form for internal use, as creams and ointments for use on the external skin and as pessaries and creams for use in the vagina. Nystatin is the preferred medication for oral use because it is very poorly absorbed from the gut into the bloodstream and so is safe to take, even in large quantities, with little likelihood of toxic side-effects. Nystatin is toxic to yeast cells by altering the integrity of the cell wall to the extent that it causes the cell to die and break down. It is also thought to inhibit Candida's conversion to the troublesome mycelial form which burrows into the gut wall and severely irritates it.

Treatment is usually begun by taking one capsule (or tablet) four times daily. approximately every six hours, as that is the period of time that Candida takes to flare up. At the same time, it is best to treat any affected skin areas by the use of another appropriate nystatin preparation. Over a period of weeks, the oral nystatin may be gradually increased to sixteen or more capsules per day (four, four times daily) but symptoms may be relieved at a lower dosage. The appropriate maintenance dosage is different for each individual and must be established after several weeks by a gradual reduction in the dose of nystatin until symptoms reoccur. Then the dosage should be increased slightly until symptoms are relieved. The maintenance dose is the minimum required to control symptoms.

Commencement of a course of nystatin at low dosage levels is important if one is to avoid the after effects of 'die-off'. Whenever there is severe Candida proliferation in the gut, large doses of nystatin cause large numbers of yeast cells to 'die-off' resulting in the release of a much larger than normal quantity of yeast metabolites which, when carried to other parts of the body in the bloodstream, cause toxic reactions which are easily recognisable as uncomfortable symptoms. On occasions, these reactions to the massive release of toxic metabolites can be quite severe but can be avoided by gradually increasing the nystatin dosage.

Nystatin is generally well tolerated by most people but may cause nausea in some individuals. Some individuals, who are very sensitive, may react to the non-active ingredients in the tablets or capsules and can tolerate only the pure powder which may be taken stirred into water. Taken this way, nystatin's bitter taste cannot be avoided but it is tolerable.

Other anti-yeast antibiotics which can be used are amphotericin (Fungilin) and ketoconazole (Nizoral). Compared with nystatin, these tend to be absorbed into the bloodstream and thus may lead to toxic side-effects especially in individuals with impaired liver function. For that reason, amphotericin and ketoconazole are generally reserved for the more stubborn cases resistant to nystatin or where there is a sensitivity to nystatin.

Common garlic, although not an antibiotic as such, is known to be inhibitory to Candida and many people have reported beneficial results after taking garlic as oil or powder.

Lactobacillus acidophilus, which is the culture bacteria used in the manufacture of yoghurt is one of the friendly bacteria which compete with yeasts in the gut. Re-establishment of the normal levels of Lactobacillus in the gut by supplementation of the diet with yogurt or *Lactobacillus acidophilus* tablets or powder has been reported to reduce the symptoms associated with Candida imbalance.

Resting of the Immune System by Avoidance of Yeast-based Foods

When the immune system is tired or unwell, recovery is assisted by rest. You cannot put your immune system to bed for a rest, but you can help by reducing its workload. The immune system is a complex one involving many organs which combine to protect the functioning body against any foreign chemicals. The compromised immune system cannot cope with what is a normal load of invading chemicals so you must attempt to relieve that load by reducing the amount of foreign chemicals entering the system.

The most common source of foreign chemicals is improperly digested foodstuffs which can be absorbed from the gut, especially if the gut lining is damaged by a chronic Candida imbalance. Digested yeast cells, either from the gut or from yeast-based foods are a major source of chemicals or metabolites which act as troublesome compounds.

One major way of reducing the load on the immune system is to reduce the amount of yeast metabolites which reach the gut. This can be done by reducing or eliminating yeast-based foods from the diet and by reducing or eliminating from the diet those foods which have a tendency to encourage yeast proliferation in the gut.

Foods employing yeast processes during their manufacture include bread, cheese, wine and beer which, with many others listed in Chapter 5, are foods to be avoided.

Identification and Avoidance of Chemical and Other Allergens

There are thousands and thousands of chemicals, foreign to our bodies, which contaminate our environment and their number and quantity appear to be increasing every day. Man-made chemicals contaminate everything with which we come in contact, including the air we breathe and the food we eat. All of these chemicals are potentially toxic when absorbed by the body and require detoxification by the immune system in order to maintain health and well-being. Therefore, each one contributes to the overall allergenic load with which the immune system has to cope.

It is possible to substantially reduce this load by avoiding exposure to chemical pollutants such as vehicle exhaust fumes, cigarette smoke and industrial pollutants, and by ensuring an adequate supply of fresh clean air and avoiding heavily polluted areas. While this may sometimes be difficult, there are ways you can reduce your contact with pollutants. When driving in heavy traffic, make sure your windows are closed. Ask your friends if they would mind not smoking in your home. If possible, avoid going out on days when air pollution levels are high. Food crop sprays, preservatives, stablisers, emulsifiers and all the other chemicals which constitute additives in processed food can be avoided by ensuring that all foodstuffs are fresh and preferably organically grown.

Foods to which you are allergic will also place an added burden on the immune system. An allergic reaction to a food is brought about by some improperly digested food (usually protein) being identified by the immune system as foreign and requiring detoxification. Sometimes, supplementation with digestive enzymes as tablets or capsules assists digestion sufficiently to ensure that the particular allergen no longer causes a reaction. Food intolerances need to be identified in order that they may be avoided so as to reduce the workload of the immune system.

Inhaled allergens (usually pollens) place an extra burden on a weakened immune system and should be avoided if possible, although that may be rather difficult. Measures can be undertaken to assist this. Stay indoors on windy days. Cleaning of the air in your office or work area by the use of air filters or negative ion generators may also help.

Avoidance of Exposure to Yeast Spores

When mould cells mature, they release into the atmosphere

millions of microscopic spores which are then carried about by the wind. These spores are inhaled along with the air and are captured in the mucous lining of nasal passages and breathing tubes. The mucous is continually being swept to the back of the nose and to the top of the windpipe, carrying the mould spores along with it. Usually, it is swallowed and thus ends up in the stomach and gut where the spores may be digested or may lead to infestation. Either way, they release mould metabolites into the gut where they can be absorbed into the bloodstream and then require detoxification by the immune system.

Avoidance of areas where the atmosphere is mouldy or musty and by cleaning up mould in damp areas can help to reduce the load on the immune system.

Mould avoidance measures are described more fully in Chapter 8.

Avoidance of Immunosuppressant Drugs

The cortisone-type medications encourage Candida proliferation by directly encouraging yeast growth and concurrently suppressing the body's immune system which is its natural defence. The immunosuppressant action is beneficial when it is used to treat an abberration of the immune system which sometimes occurs when it is unable to differentiate between native and foreign tissue and attacks some of the body's own normal chemicals. But when the ultimate aim of the treatment is to regenerate an effective immune system, these medications are detrimental and are best avoided.

Stimulation of the Immune System with Candida Extracts

Allergy extracts or 'vaccines' consist of injectable products which contain ingredients to which the patient has developed an allergic reaction. *Candida albicans* extract is derived from

Candida albicans cells and prepared in such a way that it may be injected. Minute, carefully controlled doses are injected under the skin at a rate which is designed to stimulate the immune system to respond to Candida material. The goal is to replace the unpleasant allergic reaction with a positive immune detoxification response so that symptoms no longer result from exposure to that allergen.

Aiding the Immune System by Supplementation with Vitamins and Minerals

Poor digestion and mal-absorption problems coincide with mal-absorption of vitamins and minerals. At the same time, any detoxification exercise undertaken by the immune system is a consumer of vitamins and minerals especially vitamins A, C and E and selenium.

Supplementation of the diet with extra vitamins and minerals is aimed at enhancing the recovery of the immune system to its normal functioning capacity as well as assisting it by providing it with an adequate amount of all the raw materials necessary for it to do its job. A more detailed discussion of which vitamins and minerals are required to accomplish this is contained in Chapter 7.

CHAPTER 5

The Anti-Candida Diet

Basic Dietary Guidelines

The anti-Candida diet aims to provide an easily prepared, nutritionally balanced and interesting eating plan which will restore the yeast balance in the body. For it to be successful, two food types *must* be avoided.

1 Refined Carbohydrate

Yeasts thrive and multiply on refined or simple carbohydrates. The most commonly occurring simple carbohydrate in the Western diet is cane sugar. It is used extensively as a sweetener in soft drinks, cakes, biscuits, jams, jellies, confectionery, most packaged breakfast cereals and many prepared foods. Honey contains an especially high concentration of simple sugars.

2 Yeast, Moulds and Fungi

Where a yeast imbalance exists in the body, these will further destabilise the immune system. Yeast and moulds are present in some foods as a necessary ingredient. The most obvious example is the use of baker's yeast in bread. They are also present, however, in many prepared foods such as tomato products and fruit juices and mould can appear on fresh food that is not eaten immediately. Mushrooms and champignons are, of course, fungi.

A balanced diet must provide carbohydrate, proteins, fats, vitamins and minerals. This can be achieved by a combination of the five basic food groups.

1 Cereals
2 Meats, fish, eggs, beans and lentils
3 Milk and other dairy products
4 Fruit and vegetables
5 Butter, margarine and oils

The anti-Candida diet is based on such a balanced combination with certain foods removed. It does not necessarily require a radical change of lifestyle and lends itself to adaptation of the regular family menu.

The diet is divided into three stages. The first lasts for two to three weeks when the guidelines must be followed strictly. In the second stage, which lasts for another six to ten weeks, the range and quantity of food are more flexible. The third stage is a time for expanding the diet towards a return to normal and involves careful testing of foods to establish those which should be permanently avoided. Obviously, the more closely you follow the diet, the more quickly you will regain your health.

After a period on the diet your tolerance for most foods will return. There are two reasons for this. Firstly, whilst on the diet, your immune system and your digestive system have been rested. Newly restored, these systems can now cope. Secondly, the yeast imbalance may have changed your intestine lining. With your yeast and bacteria in balance, most foods which previously caused a problem can be eaten freely.

With your health restored, the diet provides you with a weapon to use if your symptoms reappear or if you are in a stressful situation. It is wise to follow the diet if you have to use antibiotics at any time. Although the effects of Candida infection can be eliminated, the predisposition will remain and it can reoccur any time when the right formula appears.

Be aware of your own body and its vulnerabilities. You don't have to wait for symptoms to reappear. For instance, if you know a stressful time is approaching — exams, job interviews, a family party — do something about it before you begin to feel unwell. Follow Stage 1 of the diet for a couple of weeks and see how well you breeze through the crisis!

Here are some case histories of people who have suffered some of the many symptoms caused by yeast infection and infestation and have had their health restored under the anti-Candida regime outlined in this book.

Carrol is a single, professional woman aged twenty-seven. She was referred by her doctor having suffered from chronic thrush for six months. Her eating habits were fairly average. She particularly liked cheese and cakes and often ate pizza. She enjoyed wine occasionally.

She was put on the anti-Candida diet and followed it for eight weeks. By the end of the first month the thrush had disappeared completely. After another month she began experimenting with some of the foods she had been avoiding. She found that the irritation returned with high carbohydrate foods and wine.

A year later she is completely free of thrush and feeling well. If irritation does occur, she returns to the strict diet for two weeks.

Bob is a pharmacist aged forty-four. He tried unsuccessfully to lose weight over a long period of time eating only 1500 kilojoules per day on a wide range of diets. He drank a large amount of coffee: up to eight cups a day. Although he did not mention other symptoms to begin with, he also had a chronic rash on his back and suffered from swollen feet and ankles in heat.

He commenced the anti-Candida diet and after two weeks he had lost four kilos and the rash on his back had cleared. It was at this point that he first mentioned it. After twelve weeks he had lost 13.5 kilos and the problem with swelling ankles had disappeared. After twelve months he has lost a further 10 kilos and his weight is constant. Bob is still a big man but his blood pressure is normal. He returns to the strict yeast-free diet when he is under stress.

Grace is a secondary school English teacher. She is fifty-seven years old. Referred by her doctor because she was marginally overweight, she presented with a variety of symptoms. She was suffering headaches and a painful, stiff neck. She also reported halitosis and thick, foul-tasting saliva, dermatitis under her wedding ring, loose bowel movements, and nausea when waking and after meals.

Ten years ago she had a hysterectomy and she has had surgery for varicose veins three times. At the time of referral she was taking no medication. Her diet was well balanced.

She began the anti-Candida diet and after two weeks the rash under her ring had gone, and the bad breath had also disappeared. The thick, foul-tasting saliva was diminishing. After six weeks on the diet she reported that her bowels were normal and that the saliva problem had cleared. After twelve weeks she had lost a total of four kilos and was feeling much better. She tested wine and found that the foul taste in the mouth returned. Sweet and sour food brought a return of flatulance and an uncomfortable bloated feeling.

She has removed some foods permanently from her diet and uses the strict anti-Candida diet as a weapon when any of her earlier symptoms reappear. After a year, her weight is constant and seven kilos below what it was and she is a happy and healthy woman.

Christopher is a thirty-nine-year-old radio announcer. He was referred by a doctor for weight reduction but also revealed high blood pressure, headaches, bad tinea, and lethargy. He often felt bloated in the abdomen. He was very concerned about chronic sore throats which many medical tests had indicated were of no consequence.

His eating habits were poor and this seemed to be related to his work routine. He was very keen on tomato sauce and had noticed that red wine upset him.

After a month on the anti-Candida diet the sore throat and tinea had disappeared and his energy level had increased. He then proceeded to test foods and identified those he should avoid. After a year he enjoys good health and his weight is constant.

Penny is a thirty-four-year-old primary teacher. She has two children aged ten and thirteen. She was referred by her doctor because of hay fever and pre-menstrual tension and because she wanted to lose weight. She was also suffering constipation and headaches and reported pains in the stomach when pre-menstrual.

In general, her diet was well balanced with occasional indulgences of cakes and desserts. At the time she was exercising three times a week and seemed a happy and extroverted woman. She socialised often. Although she was not seriously over-weight, she expressed a desire to be a size smaller.

After two weeks on the anti-Candida diet she lost three kilos and reported no headaches. After four weeks she lost a further kilo and her period had arrived without the usual pre-menstrual symptoms. Another month later, after stress at work, she reported period pain and moodiness once again. Her weight had dropped two kilos. After four months she was maintaining her weight loss and was suffering no further trouble with her periods. The headaches and constipation had gone. She was eating most foods but was avoiding baker's yeast. She returns to the strict diet if she gains weight or has any recurrence of the earlier symptoms.

Establishing the Diet

Nutritional Balance

Because you are on a diet, even a strict one for the first two to three weeks, this does not mean that your meals and those of your family have to be bland or dull. A wide range of foods are allowed under the anti-Candida regime and the number and variety of recipes in this book indicate the range of good food which will still be available to you as well as your family and friends.

It is vital that your diet should consist of a wide variety of foods. A combination from the five basic food groups will ensure balanced nutrition. If you find you are intolerant to one particular food or food group it is essential you replace nutrients which may be lacking. For example, if milk and dairy products are a problem and must be avoided, you must pay particular attention to your calcium requirements. If one grain or cereal or one type of fruit causes a problem, the other foods within the group will usually cover any nutrient deficiencies.

Vegetarians must pay particular attention to their protein intake, especially if cheese has been part of their staple diet. Milk, ricotta and cottage cheese, and cereal proteins are important substitutes for non-meat eaters on this diet. A range of vegetarian dishes is provided in the recipe section.

Allowed Foods

Here is a list of the foods which can be eaten freely on the diet and from which you should select a balanced range from the five food groups.

Cereals (wholegrain or wholemeal)

Wheat
Rice
Oats
Barley
Corn (maize)
Millet
Buckwheat
Triticale

Protein

Meat: beef, veal, lamb, mutton, pork, rabbit
Poultry: chicken, turkey, duck, goose, quail
Fish: saltwater or freshwater, shellfish (oysters, mussels, scallops), crustaceans (crayfish, lobster, crab, prawn, shrimp)
Eggs: chicken, duck or quail

Nuts: almonds, cashews, Brazil-nuts, macadamia nuts and pecan nuts
Seeds: pumpkin, sesame and sunflower seeds, lentils, dried peas and beans

Milk and dairy products

Milk: cows', goats'
Natural yoghurt (Preferably this should be made with a culture of *Lactobacillus acidophilus*. This is available commercially.)
Cottage cheese
Ricotta cheese
Buttermilk

Vegetables

All fresh vegetables except mushrooms and champignons. Frozen vegetables as long as they are used immediately and not refrozen.

Fruits

All fruits except grapes. Check the skin of rockmelon or cantaloup for soft spots. Use melons immediately they are cut.

Butter, margarine or oils

Stocking Up

The essential ingredient of this diet is fresh food; fresh fruit and vegetables, fresh yeast-free bread and cereals, freshly cooked meat. Shop as frequently as possible and try to have food on hand for no more than three days at a time. It is vital that there is no mould or mildew on any food. Read through the recipes, choose some that appeal to you and plan your menus for the days ahead. Make sure you buy in any ingredients you have not previously had in stock.

It is best to make your own cottage cheese and yoghurt but if this is not possible buy small quantities at a time and use completely within two days of opening packages. Buy small quantities of grains and nuts and replenish stores frequently.

As you will be shopping frequently for fresh fruit and vegetables, you will be able to produce an exciting meal in minutes. Here is an example.

Soup and toasted pita bread
Brown rice and stir-fried vegetables
Barbecued meat, chicken or fish
Fresh fruit salad
or
Pancakes with strawberry spread topped with Home Made Sour Cream (p. 100)

The Freezer

When you commence the diet, set aside some time to make up stand-by meals from the list of recipes and store them in the freezer. You will then have food available when you are caught out by the arrival of unexpected guests or when you have had one of those days when you can't keep up with everything. Here are some examples.

Soup
Pancakes
Unsweetened stewed fruit
Cooked brown rice
Cooked wholemeal pasta
Wholemeal pita bread

In the refrigerator always have some of the following on hand.
Strawberry Topping (p. 119)
Mayonnaise (p. 102)

To Be Avoided

Here is a list of foods which must be avoided in Stage 1 and, in general, in Stage 2 of the diet, along with substitutes for those foods. The substitutes can be eaten quite freely.

FOODS TO AVOID	SUBSTITUTES
Bread containing baker's yeast Buns Bread rolls	Sour dough bread Pita bread (wholemeal)
Matured cheese Blue vein cheese Processed cheese (During the manufacture of cheese, moulds and bacteria are used which can affect you in the initial stages of the diet.)	Fresh cottage cheese ✓ Fresh ricotta ✓ (If possible, these should be home made.)
Fruit and vegetables which show signs of bruising or mould growth anywhere	Fresh fruits and vegetables
Mushrooms, champignons, truffles and any fungi	
Grapes	

FOODS TO AVOID	SUBSTITUTES
Dried fruits; sultanas, raisins, muscatels, dates, apricots, prunes and figs. These are high in carbohydrates and often are contaminated with yeasts and moulds during the drying process.	Fresh fruit
Peanuts and pistachio nuts which have naturally occurring moulds	Walnuts, cashews, Brazil-nuts, almonds, hazel-nuts, pecan nuts
Tomato sauce, tomato paste, tomato juice, tomato puree and dehydrated tomato	Freshly cooked tomatoes
Commercial fruit juice (It is not always possible to avoid the inclusion of mouldy fruits in production.)	Freshly squeezed juice
Pickled, smoked or otherwise processed meats and fish, including sausages, hot dogs, corned beef, pastrami and pickled fish such as herrings	
Tea, herb teas and coffee	These are allowed if limited to 3 cups per day.
Vinegar (distilled from grain, apple, wine, rice or other sources) and vinegar-containing foods such as mayonnaise, salad dressings, mustard,	Freshly squeezed lemon juice Home made dressings and sauces

FOODS TO AVOID	SUBSTITUTES
sauces (tomato, Worcestershire, barbecue), pickles, pickled vegetables, relishes, green olives and sauerkraut	
Vitamins of the B complex group (either alone or in multivitamin preparations) as they are often derived from yeast.	If vitamins are necessary use a yeast-free, sugar-free brand. This will be stated on the label.
Beer Wine, Sherry, Port or other fortified wine Brandy Champagne Cider (Alcohol breaks down in the body into simple sugars. Also, many alcoholic drinks are manufactured using yeast.)	If you are out socially after the first 2 weeks, the occasional drink of gin, vodka, whisky or rum with a low calorie mixer such as soda or dry ginger is allowed as these alcoholic drinks are distilled.
Honey and other natural sweeteners including molasses, maple syrup and brown sugar.	
Pastries, cakes, biscuits, commercial pancakes, donuts, puddings, bread rolls, scones, pies, tarts, spaghetti and other pasta, thickened soups and sauces, pizza or any other food which contains refined (white) flour. This includes refined flour made from wheat, corn, rice, or any other source.	Wholemeal pastries and scones Wholemeal pasta Yeast-free, wholemeal pancakes

FOODS TO AVOID	SUBSTITUTES
Sugar and sugar-containing foods including sweet pastries, cakes, biscuits, donuts, puddings, pies and tarts, jams, jellies, confectionery, canned fruits, cordials, soft drinks, icy poles and ice cream, fruit juice drinks. (It is essential to read the ingredient lists on the labels of all processed foods. Sugars may be listed by their proper names which include: sucrose, fructose, maltose, lactose, glucose, dextrose, mannitol sorbitol, galactose or corn syrup.)	Fresh fruit Fresh fruit juice
Spices and dried herbs (These often gather yeast and moulds in storage.)	Fresh herbs

The Stages of the Diet

Stage 1

This first stage requires complete elimination of yeast and refined carbohydrate from the diet and the restriction of complex carbohydrates and should be maintained for two to three weeks. The recipes in this book have symbols indicating the approximate carbohydrate content in each serve.

negligible or no carbohydrate

 low carbohydrates

 medium carbohydrates

Adults should have no less than ten medium serves daily and these must be spread evenly throughout the day. Children can have more, although twelve medium serves is usually adequate for their appetites. Children's diets should not have complex carbohydrates limited too severely. Although strict adherence to the plan may be difficult, it is strongly advised. Those suffering the effects of Candida infection have usually been ready to make sacrifices with the promise of renewed health as reward.

Stage 2

After two to three weeks strict observance of the diet many find they can relax the quantities as set down but stay within the guidelines. The amount of complex carbohydrate can be increased to sixteen or more serves daily depending on appetite demands. This should be followed until there is continued absence of symptoms and you feel well enough to reintroduce some of the foods eliminated.

Stage 3

Depending on the rate of recovery, on average four to six weeks for men and children, and twelve weeks for women, some of your favourite foods may now be reintroduced one at a time. For example, if one of your greatest sacrifices on this diet has been cheese, you could try some fresh block cheese one day after the initial six to twelve weeks. If you have no reaction, try some more after another five days. The period between trials can become shorter so eventually you may find you can have a formerly 'forbidden' food daily.

It would be unwise to use a compound food as a trial, such as pizza, because if your symptoms return you are faced with the problem of identifying the culprit: yeast in the crust, to-mato paste, cheese, mushrooms or the sausage meat?

When reintroducing foods to your diet you may find it easier to keep notes. If a food doesn't agree on the first trial, try some others, then a few weeks later re-test the original.

Continue to test foods progressively and over a period of time you will be able to identify those which you should avoid permanently. Apart from these foods, your diet should now be able to return to normal.

If, at any stage, your symptoms reappear, or you can anticipate a stressful time approaching, return to Stage 1 of the diet for two weeks to rest your system and restore the yeast balance once again.

All this sounds wonderful in theory but in day to day living you have to be practical. It is suggested that you be extremely careful for the first two weeks. Thus, there is no point starting this, or any other modified eating pattern two days before Christmas or a family celebration. Choose a fortnight where you can specify what you eat without facing stressful decisions.

You could suffer withdrawal in some form when you begin the diet. Symptoms may get worse, a headache might appear, you could come down with a sudden cold. This usually will only last for four days. It is wise therefore, if you work Monday to Friday, to commence the changes in your eating habits on Thursday. On Friday you may not feel a hundred per cent and if you have to, Saturday and Sunday can be spent looking after yourself. Monday will arrive and life should be looking decidedly brighter.

Menu Ideas, Socialising, Entertaining

The anti-Candida diet does not condemn you to a life as a recluse. You do not have to give up socialising, eat alone, or impose a dull and strict regime on your family. You do have to think carefully about what you eat, plan meals in advance and anticipate occasions when you may be caught out.

The recipes in this book indicate the wide range of delicious and interesting food which is available to you. Use them as a tool for restoring your own health while continuing your daily routine. Here are some menu ideas which should help you to plan and prepare in advance.

Breakfast

Freshly squeezed fruit juice
Oatmeal porridge and milk
Rice cakes and mashed banana

Half grapefruit
Pancakes with unsweetened apple
Home Made Sour Cream (p. 100)

Fresh fruit salad
Cottage cheese
Corn Bread (p. 44) and sliced tomato

Wedge of paw paw
Omelette with fresh herbs
Wholemeal Scones (p. 46) and butter or Mayonnaise (p. 102)

Light lunch

Soup
Chicken and salad sour dough sandwich
Tuna and salad in pita pocket
Omelette
Wholemeal pasta and home made Tomato Sauce (p. 102)

Fruit salad
Banana Pancakes (p. 112)
Yoghurt Fruit Dessert (p. 108)

Packed lunch

Sandwiches made with pita bread, sour dough bread or crispbreads and filled with egg, fish, chicken, or cold meat from last night's dinner. Add any salad combination: lettuce, tomato, cucumber, grated carrot, alfalfa sprouts.

Fill a container with cottage cheese and add chopped celery and parsley or mixed chunks of fruit. Have with a salad.

Luncheon party

Cucumber Soup (p. 61)
Wholemeal Scones (p. 46)

Stuffed Eggs (p. 54)
Garden Salad (p. 87)

Fruit Kebabs (p. 108)

Drinks:
Summer Fizz (p. 113)
Fruity Delight (p. 114)

After school snack

Milk or fresh fruit juice
Crispbreads with egg and Mayonnaise (p. 102)
Cottage cheese
Sliced tomato, avocado

Between meal snacks

Fruit
Freshly popped corn
Nuts
Crispbread with sliced tomato, avocado, banana

Dinner

Summer Menu:
Cucumber Soup (p. 61)
Chicken Salad with Rice (p. 83)
Yoghurt Parfait (p. 112)

Winter Menu:
Pumpkin Soup (p. 62)
Baked Snapper (p. 71)
Ratatouille (p. 96)

Dinner party

Avocado Dip (p. 49) with blanched vegetables and water
crackers or rice cracker biscuits
Salmon Mousse (p. 53)
Chicken Parcels (p. 82), Ginger Sauce (p. 101), carrot
sticks and French beans
Cheese Cake (p. 110) with berries in season

Children's party

Small meat balls on toothpicks with home made Tomato
Sauce (p. 102)
Salmon Dip (p. 48) with blanched vegetables, water crack-
ers and rice cracker biscuits
Home popped corn
Savoury Cases with Chicken Filling (p. 56)
Lamb Kebabs (p. 78)
Ice blocks (frozen pieces of fruit on icy pole sticks)
Banana ice cream (Freeze a banana and blend. It turns out
like ice cream.)
Jellied fruit juice served in orange halves
Individual jellied fruit moulds
Fruit Kebabs (p. 108)

If your child is having a party and he or she is on the anti-
Candida diet, serve traditional party food along with the food
your child is allowed. If your child is attending other parties,
you can send along a special plate of food which your child
will recognise and therefore be able to have something safe
to eat. If the wrong food is eaten the symptoms will return,
although only for a short time, and this will serve to underline
the need for continuing the diet. If no symptoms occur, this
will indicate the time has come to start relaxing the diet.

Adaptions

Your favourite recipes and those of your family can be adapted. Use home made sauces, dressings or other condiments instead of commercial brands; replace refined grains with whole grains; have fresh fruit and vegetables on hand instead of processed ones.

Adapt your usual breakfast. If you are used to having cereal, milk and sugar and a slice of toast and jam, use a yeast-free, complex carbohydrate cereal with milk and add fruit to sweeten it. Follow with toasted sour dough bread with sliced tomato.

If you're adapting one of your old recipes and it calls for breadcrumbs, remember crushed breakfast cereal, rice bran, rolled oats, ground nuts or seeds and crumbed sour dough bread will all serve the purpose.

Socialising and Travelling

When dining out either at a restaurant or at a friend's home, it is wise to take the edge off your appetite before you leave home. Some fruit and yoghurt will ease the pangs as pre-dinner nibbles are passed around containing ingredients you suspect you shouldn't have. Of course, if there are salad vegetables and dip available you can help yourself. Later, you may have to decline part of the main course or dessert. If you have had your yoghurt and fruit, you should still be quite satisfied.

If you are visiting friends, you can tell them what you should and shouldn't eat when the invitation is accepted. If you are attending a restaurant, telephone a day ahead and ask the chef if a plain grill and salad could be made available for you. Look for fresh fruit salad or another fresh fruit dish for dessert.

When travelling on a long car or bus trip, take yeast-free biscuits and bread, sandwiches and fruit, or if you have room, an insulated lunch box with salad and your favourite snack inside. Don't leave home hoping there will be the right food available when your scheduled stops occur. Invariably it won't be and you will be faced with a pie and sauce or cheese sandwich when you are extremely hungry.

6

Recipes

Note The use of salt in any of the recipes in this chapter is optional.

Bread Substitutes

Bread is probably the single most difficult food to renounce when undertaking an anti-Candida diet. However, there are a number of alternatives which can either be bought or made at home. All still contain carbohydrate so should only be consumed in moderation.

A number of yeast-free, complex carbohydrate breads are now available commercially. Sour dough bread can be found in most health food shops and Lebanese or pita bread is widely available. There are rice cakes and rice crispbreads on the market and some brands of puffed crispbread contain no yeast. Check the labels before you buy.

There are also a number of bread substitutes which can be made at home and are ideal, particularly for breakfast.

Note:
1 teaspoon = 5ml
1 tablespoon = 15ml
To measure 1 cupful, fill to 250ml on a measuring jug.

BASIC PANCAKES

1 cup wholemeal plain flour
1 egg
1 cup milk
pinch salt

Sift the flour and salt and gradually work in egg and half the milk, beat well for one minute and add remainder of milk. Allow to stand for 30 minutes to produce a lighter batter. Add sufficient quantity to a hot pan greased with butter, margarine or oil and cook both sides to a light brown colour. Serve with fruit or savoury filling. Pancakes may be frozen and served freshly thawed as a bread substitute or with a savoury filling.

Serves 4

Variation Add a mashed banana, some grated apple or 2 table-spoons of ground hazel-nuts to the batter.

BUCKWHEAT PANCAKES

1 cup buckwheat flour
1 cup maize meal
1 egg
1½ cups milk or water

Mix together the dry ingredients and stir in the egg and half the liquid until smooth. Beat well while adding the remainder of the liquid. Pour sufficient into a hot pan, greased with butter, margarine or oil and cook well on both sides. Serve hot with freshly stewed apple, apricots or peaches, or a savoury filling.

Serves 4

Variation Substitute rice or potato flour for maize meal. Add a mashed banana, a grated apple or 2 tablespoons of ground hazel-nuts to the batter mixture.

COCONUT PANCAKES ◈

1 cup coconut
1 cup soy or rice flour, or maize meal
3 teaspoons baking powder
½ teaspoon salt
2 tablespoons oil
2 cups water

Place all ingredients into a blender or food processor and blend until just mixed. Pour sufficient into a hot pan greased with butter, margarine or oil and cook both sides.

Serves **4**

POTATO PANCAKES ◈

1 tablespoon butter, margarine or oil
2 medium potatoes, cooked, mashed and still warm
1 tablespoon maize meal
pinch of salt

Stir butter or oil into potato and then add dry ingredients to provide a soft, dry consistency. Roll onto a floured surface to desired thickness. Cut into circles, prick all over and place in a hot pan greased with butter or oil and cook both sides. Serve hot as a basis for scrambled eggs or other savoury toppings or cold as a bread substitute.

Serves **4**

COTTAGE CHEESE PANCAKES ◈

1 egg
1 cup cottage cheese
1 tablespoon oil
½ cup wholemeal plain flour
¼ cup white plain flour
1 tablespoon skim milk powder
½ cup water
margarine, butter or oil for greasing pan

Beat the egg and blend in the cottage cheese and add remaining ingredients. Pour sufficient batter into a hot pan greased with butter, margarine or oil and cook both sides until brown. Serve hot or cold as for Basic and Buckwheat Pancakes (p. 40).

Serves 4

SODA BREAD (1) ◈

2 cups wholemeal plain flour
½ level teaspoon salt
½ level teaspoon bicarbonate of soda
1 level teaspoon cream of tartar
⅓ cup water
⅓ cup milk

Sift dry ingredients and make into a dough with the liquids. Quickly form into a round flat loaf and place on a greased baking tray. Cover loaf with a cake tin 15 cm deep, and bake in 230°C (450°F) oven for 30 minutes. Remove tin and leave loaf in oven for a further 10-15 minutes to brown.

Note To test if bread is cooked, tap the base of the loaf. If it sounds hollow it is ready.

SODA BREAD (2) ◈

1½ cups wholemeal plain flour
½ cup soy flour
1 teaspoon bicarbonate of soda
2 teaspoons baking powder
1½ cups buttermilk
1 egg
2 tablespoons oil

Sift dry ingredients. Add combined buttermilk, egg and oil and mix well. Turn dough onto floured board and knead lightly until smooth. Shape into a round and flatten slightly. Make 2 deep cuts in the dough to form a cross. Bake at 190°C (375°F) for 40-50 minutes.

Makes 1 loaf

SOUR DOUGH BREAD ◈

Sour dough
1½ cups whole wheat flour
3 cups water

In a bowl, combine the flour with the water and cover with cheesecloth or muslin. Leave to stand in a protected, warm place for 2 to 3 days until the mixture smells sour and has bubbles in it.

Bread

8 cups whole wheat flour
1½ cups sour dough
1½ cups water

Place flour in a bowl and rub sour dough into it as you would for scone dough. Add water slowly. Mix well with a wooden spoon, lifting the dough from the edges of the bowl. If the mixture is too moist, add a little more flour. When the dough begins to cling together, knead gently by hand for approximately 5 minutes or until it is smooth and elastic.

Shape the dough and place in an oiled bread tin. Leave overnight in a warm protected place. It will double in size so make sure your tin is large enough. Bake at 200°C (400°F) for 1 hour.

Variation Use a round loaf tin, or for rolls, cast iron gem scone irons.

CORN BREAD ◈

1 cup maize meal
½ cup soy flour
¼ cup oatmeal
¼ cup skim milk powder
1 cup milk
1 egg
½ level teaspoon salt
2 level teaspoons baking powder

Mix the dry ingredients. Mix powdered milk into the milk and mix into the dry ingredients along with the egg. Place in a greased loaf tin and bake in an oven pre-heated to 190°C (375°F) for about 30 minutes.

Makes 1 loaf

YOGHURT BREAD ◈

2 cups natural yoghurt
1½ teaspoons honey
1 heaped teaspoon bicarbonate of soda
1 teaspoon salt
1 cup kibble wheat flour, stone ground
3 cups wholemeal plain flour, stone ground

Mix yoghurt, honey and bicarbonate of soda. Add to sifted dry ingredients. Knead well. Place in an oiled bread tin or shape into a round loaf. Bake at 200°C (400°F) for 1 hour or until the bread sounds hollow when tapped.

Makes 1 loaf

DAMPER ◈

3 cups wholemeal self raising flour
2 teaspoons baking powder
1 to 1½ cups warm milk

Mix the dry ingredients and add warm milk to form a scone-type dough. Knead lightly and place in a greased loaf tin. Place in an oven pre-heated to 230°C (450°F), reset to 200°C (400°F) and bake until done, approximately 30 minutes.

POTATO CAKES ◈

2 medium potatoes, grated
1 small onion, chopped (optional)

Mix potato and onion and place sufficient quantity into a hot pan with approximately 1 tablespoon of butter, margarine or oil and cook on both sides.

Makes 6

WHOLEMEAL SCONES ◈

2 cups wholemeal self raising flour
1½ tablespoons butter or margarine
½ cup skim milk
½ cup water

Mix the flour and butter with fingertips to form a fine crumbly mixture. Mix in sufficient milk and water to make a soft dough. Roll out on a floured board and cut into scones. Place on an oiled baking tray and cook at 200°C (400°F) for 15 minutes.

Makes 8-10

BANANA LOAF ◈

1 egg
4 tablespoons butter or margarine
1 cup carrot, grated
2 ripe bananas, mashed
1½ cups wholemeal plain flour
1 teaspoon bicarbonate of soda
½ teaspoon cinnamon

Beat together the egg and margarine, fold in the carrot and bananas. Stir in the dry ingredients and mix well. Pour into an oiled loaf tin and bake in an oven at 150°C (300°F) for 1½ hours.

Makes 1 loaf

VEGETABLE LOAF ⟨M⟩

Dough

2 cups wholemeal self raising flour
½ cup natural yoghurt
¾ cup skim milk
2 teaspoons lemon juice

Blend flour and yoghurt in a blender or food processor until mixture has the consistency of fine breadcrumbs. Remove to a lightly floured board. Combine lemon juice and milk and slowly add to flour mixture. Knead well and roll out to a thickness of 2 cm.

Filling

1 medium onion, grated
1 carrot, grated
1 large potato, grated
1 tablespoon Tabouli (p. 91)
1 tablespoon fresh parsley, finely chopped
1 tablespoon fresh mint, finely chopped
1 tablespoon fresh basil, finely chopped

Combine all filling ingredients and spread evenly over the dough. Roll up as you would a Swiss roll. Moisten the top with yoghurt and sprinkle with sesame seeds or poppy seeds. Bake at 200°C (400°F) for 30 minutes or until well browned.

Serves 4

Appetisers and Entrees

Dips

Dips are ideal as an appetiser. Serve with sticks of fresh carrot or celery or with blanched beans, snow peas, broccoli, cauliflower or asparagus. Alternatively, use as a spread for pancakes or other bread substitutes.

Note To blanch vegetables, plunge into boiling water for 1-2 minutes. Rinse well in cold water and place in refrigerator until crisp.

SALMON DIP

1½ *cups ricotta cheese*
1 *170g can salmon, drained*
1 *tablespoon spring onions, chopped*
1 *teaspoon lemon juice*
pinch cayenne pepper
pinch salt

Thoroughly mix all the ingredients together and serve in a small bowl. Garnish with parsley or chopped spring onions.

Makes 2 cups

AVOCADO DIP Ⓝ

2 *avocados*
1 *large tomato*
4 *teaspoons lemon juice*
1 *tablespoon spring onions, chopped*
1 *clove garlic, crushed*

Thoroughly mix together the peeled and mashed avocado, the peeled and chopped tomato and the other ingredients and serve in a small bowl. Garnish with parsley or chopped spring onions.

Makes 2-3 cups

CUCUMBER DIP Ⓛ

1 *small cucumber*
1 *cup natural yoghurt*
2 *cloves garlic, crushed*
1 *teaspoon lemon juice*
1 *teaspoon mint, finely chopped*

Peel and grate cucumber and allow to drain. Combine other ingredients and fold in the cucumber. Serve chilled in a small bowl. Garnish with a sprig of mint.

Makes 1½ cups

SALMON AND CUCUMBER DIP Ⓝ

1 175g can salmon, drained
1 small cucumber, peeled and seeded
½ small capsicum, seeded
1 teaspoon lemon juice

Mix together all the ingredients in a blender or food processor. Pour into a small bowl and refrigerate. Serve chilled. Garnish with parsley.

Makes 1½ cups

TAHINI SPROUT DIP Ⓛ

1 cup natural yoghurt
½ cup tahini
1 teaspoon lemon juice
¾ cup alfalfa sprouts
1 clove garlic, crushed

Mix together all the ingredients and refrigerate. Serve chilled.

Makes 2-3 cups

GUACAMOLE Ⓛ

1 ripe avocado
1 small onion, finely chopped
1 tomato, finely chopped
1 tablespoon lemon juice
1 clove crushed garlic
1 tablespoon fresh coriander, finely chopped
salt

Mash avocado and combine with other ingredients. Alternatively, place all ingredients in a blender or food processor and blend until smooth. Chill.

Makes 1-2 cups

Variation Substitute basil or other fresh herbs if coriander is not available.

HUMMUS

1 cup chick peas, soaked overnight
juice of 2 lemons
2-3 cloves garlic, crushed
salt
¾ cup tahini
1 tablespoon olive oil
1 tablespoon fresh parsley, finely chopped

Boil the chick peas in fresh water for about 1 hour or until they are soft. Drain and puree either in a blender or food processor or by pressing through a sieve. Add a little of the lemon juice or some water during the blending. Add remaining lemon juice, garlic, salt and tahini and mix to a smooth paste. If it seems too thick, add a little water and mix until it has the consistency of mayonnaise. Pour into a wide, flat dish and garnish with olive oil and chopped parsley. Serve with pita bread or blanched vegetables.

Makes 2 cups

Note Although this recipe is quite high in carbohydrate, it can be eaten in Stage 2 of the diet as only small quantities are consumed at one time.

Entrees

ASPARAGUS AND PRAWN SALAD

500g asparagus
500g prawns, shelled and deveined
6-8 lettuce leaves
4 tablespoons vegetable oil
1 tablespoon olive oil
2 tablespoons lemon juice
1 tablespoon spring onions, finely chopped
salt and pepper

Cook asparagus in boiling, salted water until just tender. When ready, remove from heat and rinse under cold water. Drain well. Spoon prawns onto individual lettuce leaves or onto a large platter covered with lettuce. Arrange asparagus on top of the prawns. Combine remaining ingredients and whisk until the dressing thickens. Pour over salad and serve immediately.

Serves 4

CURRIED CAULIFLOWER

500g cauliflower
30g butter or margarine
1 medium onion, chopped
1 teaspoon fresh ginger, finely chopped or grated
1 teaspoon curry powder
½ teaspoon turmeric
1 teaspoon paprika
salt
1 teaspoon garam masala

Break the cauliflower into small pieces. Heat the butter in a large pan. Add onion and ginger and cook until the onion is transparent. Stir in the curry powder, turmeric and paprika. Add the cauliflower and cook for 5-10 minutes, stirring frequently. Add the salt, if desired, and then cover and simmer for 20 minutes or until the cauliflower is just tender. Remove lid and turn the heat up, allowing most of the liquid to evaporate. Sprinkle with garam masala and serve with steamed rice.

This is a substantial entree. It also makes an ideal lunch dish served with a salad.

Serves 4

Note Because of the spices in this recipe, it is best left until Stage 2 of the diet.

SALMON MOUSSE ◈

*½ cup hot water
3 teaspoons gelatine
220g tin red salmon
4 spring onions, chopped
¼ cup Mayonnaise (p. 102)
2 teaspoons lemon juice
black pepper
½ cup natural yoghurt*

Place hot water and gelatine in food processor and blend for 1 minute. Add undrained salmon, spring onions, mayonnaise, lemon juice and pepper and blend for further 1 minute. Add yoghurt and blend for 30 seconds. Pour mixture into individual dishes or one large mould and refrigerate until set. Turn out into a bed of crisp lettuce and serve with slices of cucumber and wedges of pita bread.

Serves 4

AVOCADO AND MELON SALAD Ⓝ

2 medium avocados, halved and stoned
1 tablespoon lemon juice
½ medium honeydew melon, seeded
¾ cup French Dressing (p. 103)

Scoop out the avocado flesh with a melon baller, place in bowl and sprinkle with lemon juice. Scoop out the melon flesh in the same way and add to the avocado balls. Chill 2 or 3 hours. Just before serving, pour over the dressing and gently toss the ingredients until well coated.

Serves 4

STUFFED EGGS Ⓛ

6 eggs, hard boiled
1 tablespoon chives, finely chopped
1 tablespoon parsley, finely chopped
2 tablespoons natural yoghurt
¼ teaspoon curry powder
2 teaspoons lemon juice
salt and pepper
cayenne pepper or parsley for garnish

Peel eggs and cut in half lengthwise. Remove yolks and mix

with the remaining ingredients. Carefully spoon back into the hollowed whites, chill and serve garnished with cayenne pepper or parsley.

Makes 12

CRAB AND CUCUMBER COCKTAIL Ⓝ

1 cucumber
1 cup celery, finely chopped
1 tablespoon chives, finely chopped
200g crab meat
juice of two lemons
black pepper
4 lettuce leaves
paprika for garnish

Remove skin from cucumber and using potato peeler, slice lengthwise into fine strips. Keep slicing until you reach the soft, seeded core. Combine with celery, chives, crabmeat, lemon juice and pepper. Arrange lettuce leaves on plates or in glasses. Spoon crab mixture onto lettuce. Garnish with paprika.

Serves 4

Variation Use salmon or some sliced white fish instead of crabmeat. Substitute sliced apple for the cucumber.

SAVOURY CASES WITH CHICKEN FILLING

Savoury bread cases
24 slices sour dough bread
¼ cup margarine or butter
1 clove garlic, crushed

Cut bread into 6cm rounds using a biscuit cutter. Press into patty tins. Melt the butter, combine with the garlic and brush bread cases lightly. Bake at 190°C (375°F) for 20 minutes or until crisp and golden brown.

Makes 24 bread cases

Chicken filling
2 cups cooked chicken, finely chopped
1 tablespoon green pepper, finely chopped
2 tablespoons celery, finely chopped
⅓ cup Mayonnaise (p. 102)
salt and pepper

Combine chicken, green pepper, and celery. Blend with mayonnaise. Season to taste with salt and pepper and chill well. Fill the bread cases with the cold chicken mixture and serve immediately.

Fills 24 bread cases

Variation Fill bread cases with Red Salmon and Spring Onion Sauce.

RED SALMON AND SPRING ONION SAUCE   ⅓ cup = ◇Ⓜ◇

3 tablespoons butter or margarine
3 tablespoons wholemeal plain flour
½ teaspoon salt
¼ teaspoon white pepper
1 cup skim milk
1 220g tin red salmon
2 tablespoons spring onions, finely chopped
2 tablespoons celery, finely chopped
2 teaspoons lemon juice
salt and pepper

Melt butter or margarine in a heavy based saucepan. Sir in flour, salt and pepper. Slowly add milk, stirring to form a smooth paste. Drain and flake red salmon and carefully fold into the sauce. Add spring onions and celery. Season with lemon juice. This is a beautifully simple sauce which has a very delicate flavour. Serve in savoury bread cases (p. 56) or pancakes.

Serves 4 on pancakes
Fills 24 bread cases

SEAFOOD COCKTAIL ◈

1 cup lettuce, chopped
1 cup celery, finely chopped
250g cooked prawns, crab, crayfish or fish fillets
1 tablespoon lemon juice
salt and pepper
4 lemon slices
4 sprigs parsley

Arrange lettuce and celery in attractive cocktail or dessert dishes. Place seafood on top and sprinkle with lemon juice and season with salt and pepper. Chill until ready to serve. Just before serving top with 2 tablespoons of Seafood Sauce and garnish with a lemon slice and sprig of parsley.

Seafood Sauce ◈

⅓ cup Mayonnaise (p. 102)
¼ cup Tomato Sauce (p. 102)
1½ teaspoons lemon juice
cayenne pepper
salt

Combine mayonnaise and tomato sauce with lemon juice, dash of cayenne pepper and salt to taste.

Variation Substitute ⅓ cup natural yoghurt for the mayonnaise.

Soups

The following selection of recipes provides a variety of soups for all seasons. Most have low or negligible carbohydrate content and so can be eaten quite freely. Soups can be served as an entree or as a lunch dish and because they can be frozen and quickly reheated, are ideal when you need to produce a quick meal.

CHICKEN STOCK ◈

1 large chicken or 500g chicken wings
3 cups hot water
1 medium carrot
1 medium onion
3 sticks celery
black pepper

Coarsely chop vegetables and combine with other ingredients in a large saucepan. Cover and simmer for 2-3 hours. Allow to cool and place in refrigerator to chill to facilitate removal of fat. Strain and use immediately or store in freezer.

BEEF STOCK ◈

500g shin beef
1 medium carrot
1 medium onion
3 sticks celery
black pepper or peppercorns

Coarsely chop vegetables and combine with other ingredients in a large saucepan. Cover and simmer for 3 hours. Allow to cool, remove fat, strain and use immediately or store in freezer.

VEGETABLE STOCK ◈

potatoes
carrots
onions
celery head
celery leaves
spinach
swede
turnip
parsnip
tomatoes
Optional:
½ lemon
black pepper
¼ cup orange juice, freshly squeezed

All or any of these vegetables in a combination would be suitable to make a vegetable stock. Chop the vegetables and cover them with water and add any extras. Bring to the boil and simmer for 20 minutes. Cover and leave to stand. When cold, strain. Puree the vegetable pulp and set aside. (This could be used to thicken soups.) The strained stock can be kept in the refrigerator and used as a base for soup as required.

CUCUMBER SOUP

1 *medium cucumber*
3 *cups chicken stock, freshly prepared*
2 *spring onions*
1 *tablespoon butter or margarine*
½ *cup white flour*
¼ *teaspoon salt*
¼ *cup yoghurt*
1 *egg yolk*
black pepper

peel cucumber first

Seed and cut cucumber into 1 inch cubes and combine with the chopped spring onions and the chicken stock in a large saucepan. Cover and simmer for 30 minutes or until the cucumber is soft. Push through a sieve and discard skins. Melt the butter or margarine in a large saucepan, stir in the flour and cook for 1 minute. Remove the pan from the heat and gradually add the cucumber stock. Stir continuously until the soup boils and thickens, add salt and pepper to taste. Combine the yoghurt and egg yolk and stir through the soup.

Serve chilled or hot, garnished with thin slices of cucumber.

Serves 4

MINESTRONE Ⓜ

½ cup borlotti beans, soaked overnight
2 cups beef stock
2 tablespoons oil
1 medium carrot, diced
2 sticks celery, sliced
1 medium onion, sliced
1 leek, sliced
2 large, ripe tomatoes, chopped
1 clove garlic, crushed
½ cup cabbage, shredded
salt and pepper

Drain beans and place in pan with 1 cup beef stock. Bring slowly to boil and simmer for 30 minutes. Heat oil in a pan and add carrots, celery and onion, cover and cook for 5 minutes. Add second cup of stock and bring to boil, add leek and tomatoes and simmer gently for 30 minutes. Add cabbage and garlic and cook gently until the vegetables are thoroughly cooked. Season to taste. Serve hot.

Serves 4

PUMPKIN SOUP Ⓛ

1 teaspoon oil
1 medium onion, finely chopped
1 cup chicken stock
500g pumpkin, peeled and diced
1 cup milk

¼ *teaspoon nutmeg, freshly grated*
salt. and pepper

Heat oil in pan, add onion, cover and cook for 10 minutes.
Add chicken stock and bring to boil. Add pumpkin and simmer
for 30 minutes. Allow to cool sufficiently to puree in a blender
or food processor to a smooth consistency. Return to pan, add
remaining ingredients and heat gently until ready to serve.
Serve with a dob of yoghurt or garnish with a sprig of parsley
or chopped chives.

Serves 4

ZUCCHINI SOUP Ⓝ

1 teaspoon oil
3 medium zucchini, thickly sliced
1 small onion, chopped
1 small potato, scrubbed and thinly sliced
2 cups chicken stock
½ teaspoon dried tarragon
salt and pepper

Heat oil in pan, and add vegetables and tarragon, salt and
pepper. Cover and cook for 10 minutes. Add stock, cover and
simmer for 20 minutes. Allow to cool sufficiently to puree in
a blender or food processor. Serve hot or cold with a dob of
yoghurt or a squeeze of lemon juice.

Serves 4

CHILLED TOMATO SOUP

500g ripe tomatoes, peeled and chopped
1 medium cucumber, chopped
1 green or red pepper, chopped
2 cups water
2 cloves garlic, crushed
2 tablespoons oil
salt and pepper

Mix all the ingredients together in a blender or food processor and puree. Serve chilled garnished with finely chopped chives.

Serves 4

TOMATO SOUP

1 kg ripe tomatoes
2 large carrots
1 stick celery
1 tablespoon oil
2 medium onions
3 cloves garlic, crushed
2 cups beef stock
1 bay leaf
1/4 teaspoon marjoram
1/4 teaspoon mixed herbs
1/2 teaspoon salt
black pepper

Heat the oil in a large saucepan and add the onion and garlic
and cook until the onion is soft. Coarsely chop the vegetables
and add to the onion and garlic. Add all the remaining ingredients and simmer gently for 45 minutes. Cool and puree
in a blender or food processor. Serve hot, garnished with a
sprig of parsley or mint or stir in a teaspoon of yoghurt.

Serves 4

ASPARAGUS SOUP ◈

500g asparagus
2 cups chicken stock
2 tablespoons butter or margarine
½ cup spring onions, chopped
2 cups celery, chopped
1 cup zucchini, chopped
2 tablespoons parsley, chopped
1 tablespoon fresh basil, chopped
or 1 teaspoon dried basil

Break the asparagus to separate the tough ends from the tender
stems. Simmer the tough ends in the chicken stock for 20 to
30 minutes. In a large pan, melt butter over low heat and add
asparagus stems, spring onions, celery and zucchini. Saute
until just tender. Do not overcook. Add parsley and basil.
Strain chicken stock and add to vegetable mixture. Pour into
a blender or food processor and blend for 1 minute or until
smooth. Reheat and serve.

Serves 4

VICHYSSOISE Ⓛ

1 cup raw potato, chopped
2 tablespoons butter
1½ cups leeks, finely sliced
½ cup onions, chopped
1 cup celery, finely chopped
1 cup chicken stock
1 cup cucumber, finely chopped
¼ cup parsley, finely chopped
½ cup watercress, finely chopped
1 teaspoon lemon juice
pinch nutmeg

Place potato in saucepan, cover with water and cook over low heat until soft. Set aside. Do not drain. Melt butter over low heat and add leeks, onions and celery. Cook gently for a few minutes. Add chicken stock and cook for about 10 minutes or until the vegetables are soft. Add remaining ingredients including the potatoes and their cooking water. Puree soup in a blender or food processor until smooth.

This soup may be served either hot or cold. If serving cold make sure it is very well chilled.

Serves 4

GARDEN SOUP Ⓛ

3 cups water
½ cup purple topped turnip, chopped
1 cup green beans, chopped
1 cup carrots, sliced
1 cup zucchini, sliced
1 cup cabbage, thinly sliced

2 tablespoons parsley, chopped
1 cup tomato, chopped
pinch thyme, rosemary and marjoram
salt

Bring water to the boil and simmer turnips, beans and carrots for 3 to 5 minutes. Add zucchini and cabbage. Simmer further 5 minutes and then add chopped parsley, tomato and herbs. Cook a little longer. Remove from heat and allow to sit for a minute before serving.

Serves 4

Seafood

Fresh fish and seafood are delicious and nutritious simply grilled or poached with some lemon juice and fresh herbs added. However, as with meat and poultry, there is always a need for variety. The following recipes indicate the wide range of seafood dishes which you can enjoy on the anti-Candida diet.

WHITING WITH GINGER

4 whiting fillets
3 tablespoons butter or margarine
1 tablespoon lemon juice
1 tablespoon fresh green ginger, grated
salt and pepper
3 medium onions, thickly sliced
3 medium tomatoes, sliced

Place fish fillets in a greased baking dish. Melt the butter or margarine, remove from heat and add the lemon juice, ginger, salt and pepper and pour over the fish. Cover with alternate layers of onion and tomato. Place in an oven pre-heated to 180°C (350°F) and bake for 25 minutes. Baste frequently. Garnish with chopped parsley or chives.

Serves 4

WHITING WITH VEGETABLE RICE ◈M◈

4 small whiting fillets
2 cups cooked brown rice
1½ cups cooked vegetables (peas, carrots, beans, celery)
salt and pepper
2 tablespoons butter or margarine

Poach the fish in water for 10 minutes. Flake the fish and combine with the other ingredients. Melt the butter in a large pan and lightly cook the rice mixture until it starts to brown. Serve immediately.

Serves 4

LEMON WHITING ◈N◈

4 fillets of whiting or other fish
black pepper
1 tablespoon butter or margarine
½ teaspoon grated lemon rind
juice of 1 lemon

Sprinkle fillets with pepper and place on grill tray. Mix together the butter, lemon juice and rind and spread half over the fish. Grill until lightly browned, turn over and spread balance of butter mixture and grill until cooked. Garnish with slices of lemon or sprigs of parsley.

Serves 4

SALMON AND ONION PANCAKE FILLING ◇Ⓛ

3 tablespoons butter or margarine
3 tablespoons wholemeal plain flour
salt and pepper
1 cup milk
1 220g tin salmon
1 medium onion, chopped
½ stick celery, chopped
2 teaspoons lemon juice

Melt the butter in a saucepan, stir in the flour and add salt and pepper. Slowly add 1 cup milk, stirring to form a smooth sauce. Drain and flake the salmon and fold into the sauce. Add the onions, celery and lemon juice. Serve with pancakes.

Serves 4

SALMON LOAF ◇Ⓛ

1 220g can salmon in brine or water
skim milk
1 medium onion, finely chopped
¼ cup lemon juice
1 green pepper, chopped
1 stick celery, chopped
pinch cayenne pepper
1 egg white
2 tablespoons oatmeal

Drain liquid from salmon and combine with skim milk to make
½ cup. Mix with remaining ingredients, place in an oiled loaf
tin and bake in an oven at 180°C (350°F) for 1 hour.

Serves 4

BAKED SNAPPER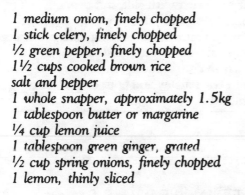

1 medium onion, finely chopped
1 stick celery, finely chopped
½ green pepper, finely chopped
1½ cups cooked brown rice
salt and pepper
1 whole snapper, approximately 1.5kg
1 tablespoon butter or margarine
¼ cup lemon juice
1 tablespoon green ginger, grated
½ cup spring onions, finely chopped
1 lemon, thinly sliced

Mix together onion, celery, green pepper, rice and salt and
pepper and stuff into the fish. Place the fish in a well greased
baking dish. Melt the butter in a saucepan, remove from heat
and add lemon juice, ginger, spring onions and salt and pepper.
Pour sauce over fish and bake in an oven pre-heated to 180°C
(350°F) for 45 minutes. Baste frequently. Place fish in a hot
serving dish, pour over juices and garnish with slices of lemon
and sprigs of parsley.

Serves 4

TROUT WITH ALMONDS

4 medium sized trout
3 tablespoons flour
black pepper
1 teaspoon salt
3 tablespoons butter or margarine
½ cup almond flakes
¼ cup lemon juice
1 tablespoon parsley, finely chopped

Coat the fish with flour seasoned with salt and pepper. Heat half the butter in a pan and cook the trout until brown. Remove and keep warm. Heat the remaining butter until foaming, add the almonds and cook until golden brown. Add the lemon juice and, stirring continuously, allow most of the liquid to boil away. Stir in the parsley and pour over the trout. Garnish with flaked almonds.

Serves 4

TUNA STUFFED PEPPERS

4 green peppers, halved and seeded
1 medium onion, chopped
1 teaspoon butter or margarine
2½ cups cooked brown rice
1 cup cottage cheese
½ cup Tomato Sauce (p. 102)
½ teaspoon thyme
1 tablespoon lemon juice
1 small can tuna, drained

Blanch the pepper halves in boiling water for 5 minutes.

Drain. Saute the onion in the butter until golden brown and add to the rice with the cottage cheese, tomato sauce, thyme, lemon juice and tuna. Fill the pepper halves with the rice mixture. Bake in an oven at 180°C (350°F) for 30 minutes.

Serves 4

PROVENCALE FISH CASSEROLE Ⓝ

2 tablespoons butter or margarine
1 clove garlic, crushed
1 medium onion, finely chopped
1 green pepper, sliced
1 red pepper, sliced
2 small zucchini, sliced
1 cup fish stock or water
500g white fish
2 ripe tomatoes, very finely chopped
1 tablespoon celery leaves, finely chopped
2 tablespoons fresh parsley, coarsely chopped
1 teaspoon fresh oregano, basil and thyme
juice of 1 lemon

Melt butter and add garlic and onion. Cook over low heat until the onions are softened. Add peppers, zucchini and stock. Cook for 2 minutes and then add fish, cut into small pieces. Simmer until fish is cooked through. Add tomatoes, celery leaves and herbs and stir gently for another 2 to 3 minutes. Pour over lemon juice and serve immediately with rice or potatoes.

Serves 4

PRAWN KEBABS ◇Ⓝ

1kg fresh prawns, shelled and deveined
2 medium onions, finely chopped
1 cup lemon juice
3 bay leaves
pinch cumin
3 large tomatoes, quartered
2 large green peppers

If the prawns are very large cut them into bite size pieces. Place them in a dish and cover with the onions and lemon juice. Add bay leaves and cumin and marinate for at least 1 hour. Thread the prawns, tomato pieces and squares of green pepper onto skewers or satay sticks. Brush lightly with oil and grill or barbecue. Serve with slices of lemon.

Serves 4

Variation Replace the prawns with scallops or fish fillets cut into small pieces.

FISH AND POTATO HOTPOT ◇Ⓜ

2 tablespoons oil
1 medium onion, sliced into rings
3 medium potatoes, thinly sliced
1 tablespoon wholemeal plain flour
500g fresh tomatoes, roughly chopped
1½ teaspoons salt
black pepper
500g fish fillets
1 tablespoon parsley, finely chopped

flounder or Cod
delicious!
Can use 4 units
canned whole
tomatoes

Heat the oil in a large heavy frying pan with a lid. Add the onion and potatoes and cook gently for 10 minutes. Turn occasionally during cooking. Stir in the flour, then add the tomatoes, salt and pepper. Cover and cook until the potatoes are almost tender, about 20 minutes.

Place the fish on top of the potatoes, cover and cook further 15-20 minutes or until the fish is cooked. Garnish with chopped parsley and serve with green vegetables.

Serves 4

Meats and Poultry

When beginning this diet, it is best to keep to plainly cooked meats. Grilled steak or chops, roast beef, lamb, chicken, turkey or pork are all most suitable. This does not mean that the food has to be boring. Season your lamb chops with a squeeze of lemon juice and some fresh herbs. Marinate your chicken in yoghurt, lemon juice and black pepper. You can also add interest to your meals with a variety of vegetables. However, there will come a time when you will want to do more than simply grill or roast.

The recipes in this section will be useful if you are entertaining, cooking for a family, or looking for something to do with cheaper cuts of meat.

You can also adapt your own favourite recipes. Remove any wine, vinegar or vinegar based products. Replace processed foods with fresh ones and avoid sugar or other refined carbohydrates.

HAMBURGERS ◈

500g lean ground beef
1 medium carrot, grated
4 spring onions, finely chopped
1 green pepper, finely chopped
1 egg, beaten
1 tablespoon Tomato Sauce (p. 102)
salt and pepper

✓
*delicious, can
be made + frozen*

Combine all the ingredients, form into patties and cook on
a barbecue or grill. Serve immediately.

Makes 4

IRISH STEW Ⓛ

1 cup water
500g boned lamb, cubed
1 large potato, cubed
2 medium carrots, chopped
1 large onion, sliced
100g green beans, chopped
1 clove garlic, crushed
1 bay leaf
1 tablespoon mixed fresh herbs (rosemary, mint, parsley, oregano)
2 tablespoons cornflour
extra ½ cup water

Bring water to the boil. Add lamb, vegetables and herbs. Cook over low heat until the meat is tender (1-1½ hours). Combine cornflour with the extra water and add to meat and vegetables. Stir until the sauce thickens. Serve immediately.

Serves 4

LAMB KEBABS Ⓛ

500g lamb, cubed
2-3 onions, thickly sliced
1 green pepper, cut into bite-size pieces
1 large zucchini, sliced
2-3 tomatoes or 1 punnet cherry tomatoes

Marinade
2 tablespoons lemon juice
½ cup olive oil

1 tablespoon fresh rosemary or mint
1 clove garlic, crushed

Combine marinade ingredients and pour over cubed lamb. Allow to marinate for at least 3 hours. Thread meat and vegetables onto skewers or satay sticks. Grill or barbecue the kebabs, basting frequently. Serve on a bed of rice. Heat the remaining marinade in a small saucepan and pour over the kebabs. Garnish with finely chopped fresh parsley.

Variation This marinade is also suitable for chicken or pork.

BEEF POT ROAST
Vegetables   Ⓜ   Meat   Ⓝ

2 tablespoons butter or oil
2 onions, sliced
1kg piece beef topside
3 cups water
2 bay leaves
sprig of thyme
2 large potatoes, sliced
3 medium carrots, sliced
1 cup peas
3 tablespoons Tomato Sauce (p. 102)

Heat butter or oil in a large pan. Add onions and meat and brown all over. Add water and herbs. Cover and simmer for about 3 hours or until the meat is tender. Add vegetables and cook for further 20 to 30 minutes. Remove meat and vegetables to a warmed serving dish. Boil stock with the tomato sauce until it is reduced to about 1 cup. Slice meat and pour sauce over meat and vegetables.

Serves 8

STIR FRY KIDNEYS Ⓝ

2 tablespoons butter or margarine
1 teaspoon fresh rosemary
1 teaspoon fresh marjoram
500g lambs' kidneys
1 green pepper, sliced
1 onion, sliced
2 stalks celery, sliced

Melt butter and add herbs. Slice kidneys very finely and add to the pan with green pepper, onion and celery. Stir fry for 3 to 5 minutes. Season with freshly ground black pepper and serve.

Serves 4

CHICKEN YOGHURT Ⓛ

4 large chicken breasts, boned
2 spring onions, sliced lengthwise
1 cup natural yoghurt
1 clove garlic, crushed
1 tablespoon parsley, finely chopped
¼ teaspoon chilli powder
¼ teaspoon cinnamon
¼ teaspoon ginger
1 teaspoon salt

Arrange the chicken breasts and onions in a baking dish. Combine the remaining ingredients and pour over the chicken and allow to marinate for several hours. Place in an oven, preheated to 180°C (350°F) and bake for 1½ hours.

Serves 4

ROAST CHICKEN WITH ORANGE

2 oranges
1 medium chicken
1 clove garlic
3 tablespoons oil

Juice one orange and put the juice aside. Prepare the chicken and rub the outside skin with the orange rind. Stuff the chicken with the other orange, quartered, and the garlic clove. Brush the outside with the oil and bake for 1 hour at 180°C (350°F). Pour over the orange juice and bake for a further 45 minutes.

Serves 4

CHICKEN CROQUETTES

1½ tablespoons butter, margarine or oil
2 tablespoons wholemeal plain flour
1 cup skim milk
2 cups cooked chicken, chopped

Melt the butter and stir in the flour and cook over a low heat for 1 minute. Remove from heat and mix in the skim milk and cook until thick. Spread the chopped chicken on a large plate and pour over the hot sauce. Allow to cool and then chill well. Form into croquettes and bake in an oven, pre-heated to 180°C (350°F) until crisp and brown.

Serves 4

CHICKEN RISOTTO ◈

1 tablespoon oil
1 clove garlic, crushed
1 cup cooked chicken, chopped
½ each of green, red and yellow pepper, chopped
2 tomatoes, chopped
½ teaspoon salt
black pepper
1 cup brown rice, cooked

Heat the oil in a pan and lightly cook the garlic, chicken, peppers and tomatoes. Add a little water and the salt and pepper and cook until vegetables are soft, stirring frequently. Add the hot, cooked rice and serve. Garnish with parsley.
Serves 4

CHICKEN PARCELS ◈

1 cup fresh apricots
2 tablespoons crushed pecan nuts
½ cup natural yoghurt
1 teaspoon fresh thyme
black pepper
4 chicken fillets
4 sheets wholemeal filo pastry
oil or butter for pastry

Combine apricots, nuts, yoghurt, thyme and pepper. Spread mixture evenly over fillets which have been flattened with a mallet. Roll up and place each one on a sheet of filo which has been lightly brushed with butter or oil. Fold into parcels and place on a greased baking tray. Bake at 200°C (400°F) for 45 minutes.
Serves 4

Salads and Vegetables

Fresh food is a vital part of this diet and so salads and vegetable dishes are ideally suited as snacks, accompaniments or as whole meals. The following collection of recipes includes a range of dishes for these different requirements. This section will be particularly useful for those who prefer or enjoy vegetarian food. If possible, shop for fresh fruit and vegetables every few days in order to ensure that they are mould and yeast free.

Main Courses

CHICKEN SALAD WITH RICE ◇

1 corn cob
1 cup cooked brown rice
2 cups lean chicken, chopped
½ cucumber, sliced
1 medium onion, finely chopped
½ green pepper, finely sliced
4 tablespoons French Dressing (p. 103)
½ cup Yoghurt Dressing (p. 104)
1 tablespoon chives, finely chopped

Cook corn cob and remove kernels with a sharp knife. Combine all ingredients, except chives, mix gently and chill before serving. Garnish with chopped chives.

Serves 4

PRAWN AND AVOCADO SALAD ⟨L⟩

1kg cooked fresh prawns
2 avocados, balled or diced
2 medium carrots, cut into strips
1 small lettuce or Chinese cabbage, finely shredded
1 spring onion, finely chopped
2 sticks celery, cut into strips
1 tablespoon roasted sesame seeds
1 cup French Dressing (p. 103)

Combine all the ingredients in a large bowl, toss lightly and chill well before serving.

Serves 4

ORIENTAL SALAD

1 cup bean or alfalfa sprouts
1 cup cooked brown rice
2 sticks celery, finely sliced
2 cups cooked lean chicken or pork
½ cup toasted almonds
3 spring onions, finely chopped
1 medium carrot, grated
½ green pepper, chopped
¾ cup French Dressing (p. 103)

Combine all ingredients in a large bowl, toss lightly and chill well before serving. Garnish with chopped parsley.

Serves 4

MACARONI SALAD ◈Ⓜ

2 cups cooked macaroni
½ medium cucumber, sliced
2 medium tomatoes, coarsely chopped
2 sticks celery, sliced
2 cups cooked cold lean meat or chicken
½ cup French Dressing (p. 103)

Combine the ingredients in a large bowl, toss lightly and chill
well before serving on a bed of lettuce. Garnish with chopped
parsley.

Serves 4

CHICKEN SALAD WITH GINGER DRESSING ◈Ⓛ

2 tablespoons butter or margarine
1 tablespoon fresh ginger, grated
1 clove garlic, crushed
4 chicken fillets
2 tablespoons water
1 lettuce
1 cup Chinese cabbage, finely sliced
½ cup red cabbage, finely sliced
2 tablespoons parsley, finely chopped
1 cup celery, finely chopped
2 tablespoons spring onions, finely chopped
2 tablespoons sesame seeds (optional)
¼ cup Ginger Dressing (p. 105)

Melt butter over low heat, add ginger and garlic and allow to soften. Add chicken, which has been cut into small pieces, and toss gently until the chicken changes colour. Place salad vegetables into a bowl and add hot chicken. Pour ginger dressing over salad immediately and toss. Top with toasted sesame seeds.

Serves 4

Variation Other crunchy salad vegetables can be added or substituted. Turkey or white fish can be substituted for the chicken.

FISH SALAD ◈

1 *lettuce or some mixed salad greens (spinach, watercress,
endive)*
2 *medium carrots, grated*
1 *green pepper, diced*
1 *cup celery, finely sliced*
3 *radishes, finely sliced*
4 *fillets fish, cooked and well chilled*
½ *cup Mayonnaise (p. 102)*
1 *cup cold cooked rice*
juice of 1 lemon

Arrange lettuce or other greens on a platter or on individual plates. Combine remaining salad vegetables and spoon over lettuce. Slice fish, mix with the mayonnaise and add the rice.

Toss lightly with the vegetables and squeeze lemon juice over the whole dish.

Serves 4

Variation Add some fresh herbs to the mayonnaise.
Use Avocado Dressing (p. 105) or Herb Dressing (p. 106) instead of mayonnaise.

GARDEN SALAD Ⓝ

Arrange this dish on individual plates. It makes a good lunch dish on a hot day.

1 bunch watercress
2 tomatoes
1 cucumber
2 carrots
2 sticks celery
500g asparagus, cooked and well chilled
4 hard boiled eggs, halved
1 cup Mayonnaise (p. 102)
fresh parsley, chives, dill, basil or other herbs, finely chopped

Arrange watercress on plates. Cut tomatoes into wedges, and slice cucumber, carrots and celery into strips. Place these, with the asparagus and eggs, around a central well on the plate. Spoon a tablespoon or more dressing into the centre of the plate and sprinkle with fresh herbs.

Serves 4

BEEF SALAD ◇L◇

This dish is a good way of using the leftovers from last night's roast!

1 lettuce
1 cup alfalfa sprouts
1 cup lean beef, sliced into strips
1 cup carrot, grated
4 radishes, finely sliced
1 cup snow peas
½ cucumber, peeled and sliced
½ cup French Dressing (p. 103)

Make a bed of lettuce on each plate. Sprinkle with alfalfa sprouts. Combine beef with remaining ingredients and toss in French dressing. Spoon over lettuce and sprouts.

Serves 4

POTATO AND CABBAGE CASSEROLE ◇M◇

cabbage leaves, blanched for 2 minutes or until pliable
2 large onions, sliced
500g cabbage, shredded
2 large apples, peeled and sliced
4 large potatoes, boiled and sliced
1 cup cottage cheese
salt and pepper

Line a casserole dish with blanched cabbage leaves and add the layers of onion, cabbage, apple and potato. Cover with cottage cheese and sprinkle with salt and pepper. Repeat layers finishing with a layer of potato. Cover and cook at 180°C (350°F) for 40 minutes. Remove cover and continue cooking until potatoes are browned.

Serves 4

SPINACH AND RICOTTA FLAN Ⓝ

1 bunch spinach, chopped
2 eggs
¼ cup skim milk powder
1½ cups ricotta cheese
½ cup tomato juice, freshly prepared
2 tablespoons parsley, chopped
black pepper
2 medium onions, sliced

Gently boil the spinach for 5 minutes, drain and cool. Beat together the eggs, milk powder, ricotta cheese, tomato juice, parsley and pepper in a blender or food processor until smooth. Oil a small casserole dish and line with spinach leaves and pour in the egg and ricotta mixture. Cook onions in a little water until soft and arrange on the egg and ricotta mixture. Bake in an oven heated to 150°C (300°F) for 45 minutes.

Serves 4

CABBAGE AND CHEESE ROLL ◆Ⓜ

2 tablespoons butter or margarine
2 medium onions, finely chopped
¼ fresh cabbage, finely sliced
1 teaspoon carraway seeds
salt and pepper
2 hard boiled eggs, chopped
3 tablespoons cottage cheese
4-6 sheets wholemeal filo pastry
oil or butter for pastry

Melt butter in a large pan. Add onions and cook gently until they soften. Add cabbage and cook for further 3 minutes. Mix in carraway seeds and season with salt and pepper. Remove from heat. Fold in chopped eggs and cottage cheese.

Brush pastry sheets with oil, butter or margarine and place one on top of the other. Place cabbage mixture at one end of pastry and roll up. Seal edges and place on a greased oven proof tray. Bake at 180°C (350°F) for 30 minutes.

Serves 4

LENTIL CURRY ◆Ⓜ

1½ cups brown lentils
1 tablespoon butter or oil
2 onions, finely chopped
2 teaspoons curry powder
½ teaspoon turmeric
500g broccoli
500g cauliflower
juice of 1 lemon

Simmer lentils in boiling water until just tender. Drain. Melt butter over low heat and cook onions until they soften. Add spices and cook for a further 2-3 minutes. Add lentils and 1 cup of water. Bring to boil and add vegetables and lemon juice. Cook for 5-10 minutes stirring occasionally. Serve with steamed brown rice.

Serves 4

Accompaniments

TABOULI (M)

¼ cup cracked wheat (bulgur)
½ cup boiling water
½ cup spring onions, finely chopped
1 cup parsley, finely chopped
1 tablespoon fresh mint, finely chopped
1 small green pepper, finely chopped
2 tomatoes chopped
1 cup celery, chopped
2 tablespoons olive oil
2 tablespoons lemon juice

Cover cracked wheat with boiling water and let stand for 2 hours. Drain through a strainer. Combine with vegetables and herbs. Add oil and lemon juice and allow to stand for 1 hour.

ORANGE COLESLAW ◇Ⓛ

2 oranges, peeled and segmented
½ cabbage, finely shredded
1 green pepper, finely sliced
1 red pepper, finely sliced
2 teaspoons lemon juice
½ teaspoon lemon rind, grated
1 cup Mayonnaise (p. 102)

Combine all the ingredients in a large bowl and chill well
before serving.

CUCUMBER SALAD ◇Ⓝ

2 medium cucumbers
1 cup celery, chopped
1 cup cold, cooked lean meat, chicken or fish, chopped
½ cup radish, chopped
½ cup French Dressing (p. 103)

Cut cucumbers lengthwise, take out some of the pulp and
combine with other ingredients to use as stuffing for the cucumber cases. Garnish with a sprig of parsley.

COLESLAW ◇Ⓛ

2 carrots, grated
½ cabbage, finely shredded
½ cup spring onions, finely chopped
1 red apple, finely chopped
1 cup fresh pineapple, finely diced
1 teaspoon lemon juice

½ cup toasted almonds
½ cup Yoghurt Dressing (p. 104)

Combine all the ingredients in a large bowl and chill well before serving.

CURRIED RICE SALAD ◈

2 tablespoons oil
2 teaspoons lemon juice
3 teaspoons curry powder
1 cup cooked brown rice
1 medium red apple, chopped
¼ cup walnuts, chopped
½ cup red or green pepper, finely sliced

Mix together the oil, lemon juice and curry as the dressing. Pour over the rice while still warm and mix well. Allow to cool and add the other ingredients and toss lightly. Serve well chilled.

TOMATO SALAD WITH GINGER ◈

4 medium tomatoes, coarsely chopped
1 small onion, finely chopped
1 teaspoon fresh ginger, finely chopped
2 tablespoons lemon juice
1 tablespoon chives, finely chopped
2 tablespoons parsley, finely chopped

Combine all ingredients except parsley, mix gently and chill before serving. Garnish with the chopped parsley.

TOSSED SALAD Ⓝ

1 *clove garlic*
1 *medium lettuce*
6 *spring onions, finely sliced*
½ *green pepper, finely sliced*
½ *red pepper, finely sliced*
4 *medium tomatoes, chopped coarsely*
1 *cucumber, sliced*
½ *cup French Dressing (p. 103)*

Rub a wooden bowl with the clove of garlic. Break up the lettuce and combine with spring onions and toss. Arrange peppers, tomato and cucumber on top and add the French dressing.

POTATO SALAD Ⓜ

4 *medium potatoes, cooked and diced*
1 *small onion, finely chopped*
1 *stick celery, sliced*
1 *cup cooked fresh peas*
½ *teaspoon mustard powder*
black pepper
2 *tablespoons parsley, finely chopped*
1 *cup Yoghurt Dressing (p. 104)*

Combine all the ingredients in a large bowl, toss lightly and chill well before serving.

TOMATO RICOTTA ◈

2 tablespoons chives, finely chopped
½ teaspoon salt
1 cup ricotta cheese
4 large tomatoes, halved

Blend the chives, ricotta cheese and salt and pepper and pile
onto tomato halves to give stuffed tomato appearance. Serve
on a bed of lettuce.

ZUCCHINI IN TOMATO SAUCE ◈

3 medium tomatoes, chopped
1 clove garlic, crushed
½ teaspoon basil
black pepper
8 small zucchini, thickly sliced

Place the tomatoes in a saucepan with the garlic, basil and
pepper and cook until soft. Mash the tomato mixture, add the
zucchini and cook until soft. Serve hot as an accompaniment
to a meat dish.

HOT POTATO SALAD ◇Ⓜ

3 medium potatoes, chopped coarsely
1 medium onion, finely chopped
1 red pepper, finely chopped
1 green pepper, finely chopped
1 stick celery, finely chopped
1 medium carrot, grated
½ cup Mayonnaise (p. 102)
black pepper

Cook potatoes until tender and mix with the other vegetables. Place in an oiled casserole dish, pour over the mayonnaise and cook in an oven at 180°C (350°F) for 20 minutes.

RATATOUILLE ◇Ⓝ

½ tablespoon oil
1 clove garlic, crushed
1 green pepper, seeded and cut into rings
1 small eggplant, sliced
2 medium onions, sliced
2 zucchini, sliced
2 medium tomatoes, sliced

Heat the oil in a large pan and add the garlic, pepper, eggplant, onion and zucchini. Cover and simmer for 10 minutes, add tomato and simmer for a further 10 minutes uncovered.

POTATOES AND ONIONS ◇L

3 *large potatoes, thinly sliced*
1 *large onion, sliced into rings*
¾ *cup skim milk*
black pepper

Oil a shallow casserole dish and layer potatoes and onions.
Pour over the skim milk, sprinkle with pepper and cook in
an oven at 180°C (350°F) for 1½ hours.

BEANS AND TOMATOES

1 *tablespoon oil*
2 *medium onions, sliced into rings*
4 *medium tomatoes, chopped*
2 *cloves garlic, crushed*
½ *teaspoon fresh basil*
1 *bay leaf*
black pepper
1½ *cups cooked kidney beans*

Add the oil to a pan and cook onion rings, add tomatoes and
garlic and cook until mixture is smooth. Add the basil, bay
leaf and pepper. Drain and add the beans, cover, and simmer
for 20 minutes. Garnish with a sprig of parsley.

SPROUTS

Sprouts are an extraordinarily versatile and nutritious vegetable. They can be grown in any climate all year round, are
high in protein and vitamins, especially C, and require little
cooking or preparation. They are also delicious! Use them in
salads, sandwiches and other snacks as well as in soups and
stir-fried dishes. Mung bean sprouts, alfalfa, clover, fenugreek
and lentil are among the most commonly used and easiest to
sprout. Each has its own flavour.

How to sprout your seeds

Successful sprouting depends on the right combination of
temperature, moisture and light. The seeds must be allowed
to swell, burst their shells and start to grow. This requires
relative darkness so the best spot for your sprouting container
is in a cupboard that is not exposed to the light too frequently.

1 Use a wide mouthed, 1 litre jar.

2 Use ½ cup of medium sized seeds (e.g. mung bean) or 1
  tablespoon small seeds (e.g. alfalfa).

3 Rinse the seeds well, place in the jar and cover with lukewarm water. Allow to soak overnight. Drain.

4 Cover the lip of the jar with a piece of cheesecloth or some
  nylon stocking. Store in a dark place. Lay jar on its side.

5 Each morning, rinse and drain seeds, and then shake the
  jar well. Continue this process for 2-5 days.

6 When the seeds are well sprouted, place in the sunlight for
  a day to allow green colour to develop.

7 Store sprouts in the refrigerator.

Sauces and Dressings

Most sauces have a medium to high carbodydrate content so are not ideal as constituents of the anti-Candida diet. However, if used only in small quantities as a dressing for a dish they will not contribute a large amount of carbohydrate to the overall diet, although it is best to leave them until Stage 2.

WHITE SAUCE

1 cup skim milk
2 tablespoons cornflour
salt and pepper

Make a thin paste of the cornflour and a small amount of the milk. Bring the balance of the milk almost to the boil. Add the paste and beat well. Add the salt and pepper.

Makes 1 cup

ALTERNATIVE WHITE SAUCE

1½ tablespoons butter
1 tablespoon wholemeal plain flour
1 cup skim milk
salt and pepper

Melt the butter in a small saucepan, stir in the flour and cook for 2 minutes. Remove from heat and slowly add milk, stirring continuously. Bring to the boil while stirring and boil until the sauce thickens to the desired consistency.

Either of these sauces can be used as a basis for various sauces by the addition of finely chopped chives, parsley, mint or sauteed onions.

Makes 1 cup

YOGHURT SAUCE

1 cup natural yoghurt
½ tablespoon cumin
1 tablespoon lemon juice
black ground pepper

Mix together all the ingredients and refrigerate until required. Yoghurt sauce is suitable for use as a dressing for a cold salad such as potato salad.

Makes 1 cup

HOME MADE SOUR CREAM

1 cup cottage cheese
½ cup natural yoghurt

Combine the ingredients in a blender or food processor until smooth. Used as a substitute for sour cream, on hot potatoes with a sprinkling of chopped cooked bacon.
    This is also delicious served with fresh fruit.

Makes 1½ cups

GINGER SAUCE ◈

2 tablespoons butter or margarine
2 onions, finely chopped
1 clove garlic, crushed
1 teaspoon fresh ginger, grated
2 teaspoons lemon juice

Melt butter and add onions and garlic. Simmer until the onions are soft. Stir in ginger and lemon juice.
   This sauce is very good with fish or steamed vegetables.

Makes 1 cup

TARTARE SAUCE ◈

This recipe is a good example of the way traditional favourites can be adapted to the anti-Candida diet.

1 cup Mayonnaise (p. 102)
2 tablespoons spring onions, finely chopped
2 teaspoons lemon juice
1 tablespoon fresh tarragon, finely chopped (if available)
1 tablespoon fresh dill, finely chopped

Combine all ingredients in a bowl and mix.

Makes 1 cup

TOMATO SAUCE ◈

This sauce can be used as an alternative to tomato paste as well as a topping for meat or vegetables. It can be stored in air tight jars in the refrigerator for a short time or frozen in small amounts.

1 tablespoon olive oil
1 large onion, finely chopped
2 cups fresh tomatoes, chopped
1 clove garlic, crushed
1 teaspoon fresh basil, oregano, and rosemary, finely chopped
1 bay leaf
1 tablespoon fresh parsley, finely chopped
salt

Heat oil and add onions. Cook gently until they soften. Add tomatoes, garlic and herbs and stir well. Add salt if desired. Cook over low heat until the tomatoes become very soft and mushy. Puree in a blender or food processor.

Makes 3 cups

MAYONNAISE ◈

2 egg yolks
½ teaspoon salt
2 teaspoons lemon juice
½ teaspoon mustard powder
black pepper
1 cup oil

Place egg yolks, salt, lemon juice, mustard and pepper in a mixing bowl and whisk until smooth. Ensure the oil is at room temperature and slowly add to the egg mixture drop by drop whisking continuously. As the mixture thickens, the oil may be added more quickly.

Makes 1 cup

COTTAGE CHEESE DRESSING Ⓝ

1 cup cottage cheese
¾ cup Home Made Sour Cream (p. 100)
1 clove garlic, crushed
2 teaspoons lemon juice
1 teaspoon mustard powder
½ teaspoon salt
black pepper

Place all the ingredients in a blender or food processor and blend until smooth. Serve chilled. This dressing may be used as a substitute for mayonnaise.

Makes 1¾ cups

FRENCH DRESSING Ⓝ

2 tablespoons oil
2 tablespoons lemon juice
½ teaspoon mustard powder
1 clove garlic, crushed
¼ teaspoon black pepper

Place all ingredients in a screw top jar and shake well. Serve chilled.

Makes ½ cup

YOGHURT DRESSING ◇Ⓛ

½ cup natural yoghurt
½ cup oil
2 tablespoons lemon juice
¼ cup chives, finely chopped
¼ cup parsley, finely chopped
1 clove garlic, crushed
½ teaspoon mustard powder
½ teaspoon salt
black pepper

Place all ingredients in a blender or food processor and blend until smooth. Transfer to a jar and refrigerate until serving.

Makes 1½ cups

CUCUMBER DRESSING ◇Ⓛ

1 cup natural yoghurt
4 teaspoons lemon juice
1 cup cucumber, coarsely grated
1 teaspoon parsley, finely chopped
black pepper

Combine all the ingredients in a jar and shake. Serve chilled as a salad dressing, as a dip for blanched vegetables, or on baked jacket potatoes.

Makes 2 cups

AVOCADO DRESSING ◇L◇

1 ripe avocado
1 clove garlic, crushed
1 tablespoon lemon juice
salt
1 tablespoon fresh mixed herbs

Place all ingredients in a blender or food processor. Blend for
1 minute or until dressing is smooth. Mayonnaise can be added
for a thinner dressing.

Makes 1 cup

GINGER DRESSING ◇N◇

½ cup olive oil
¼ cup lemon juice
1 teaspoon fresh ginger, grated
1 clove garlic, crushed

Combine all ingredients in a bowl and mix thoroughly.

Makes ¾ cup

HERB DRESSING

½ cup Mayonnaise (p. 102)
1 tablespoon fresh parsley, finely chopped
1 tablespoon fresh chives, finely chopped
1 tablespoon fresh dill, finely chopped
2 tablespoons lemon juice
2 tablespoons olive oil

Combine mayonnaise and fresh herbs. Thin dressing to desired consistency using lemon juice and olive oil. Any combination of fresh herbs can be used for this dressing.

Makes ¾ cup

Desserts

Most dessert recipes are **high** in carbohydrate because most contain sugar. For that reason, the ideal dessert is a serve of fresh fruit. However, for that special occasion or for extra interest, the following recipes may be used.

FRUITY PANCAKES

2 large cooking apples, sliced
1 cup skim milk
3 eggs
½ cup wholemeal plain flour
2 teaspoons vanilla essence

Place the apple slices in an oiled pie dish or casserole dish. Combine the remaining ingredients in a blender or food processor and blend until smooth. Pour over apple and bake in an oven pre-heated to 180°C (350°F) for 40 minutes. Serve with Home Made Sour Cream (p. 100).

Serves 4

Variation Substitute fresh apricots, peaches, pears or strawberries.

FRUIT SORBET

2 cups fresh strawberries, apricot, peach or other fruit, chopped
2 cups carrot, finely sliced
1 tablespoon lemon juice

Cook carrot until soft. Stew fruit until soft. Combine in a blender or food processor and blend until smooth. Add lemon juice and freeze in a casserole dish, stirring frequently to break up the ice crystals.

Serves 4

YOGHURT FRUIT DESSERT

2 cups natural yoghurt
4 passionfruit
1 cup fresh pineapple pieces
2 bananas, sliced

Combine all the ingredients in a bowl and stir together well. Serve chilled in individual fruit bowls.

Serves 4

FRUIT KEBABS

2 oranges
3 bananas

1 *punnet strawberries or other berries*
2 *red apples*
½ *honeydew melon*
¼ *cup orange juice, freshly squeezed*
1 *teaspoon fresh ginger, grated*
1 *tablespoon lemon juice*

Peel and chop fruit into bite size pieces. Thread alternately onto skewers. Combine remaining ingredients and pour over kebabs. Allow to marinate for 1 hour. These can be eaten as they are or grilled or barbecued. Top with fresh cream or yoghurt.

Serves 4

RICOTTA AND FRUIT TART

Wholemeal pastry
1 *cup wholemeal plain flour*
½ *cup wholemeal self raising flour*
1 *teaspoon baking powder*
2 *tablespoons butter or margarine*
1 *cup iced water*
2 *teaspoons lemon juice*

Combine dry ingredients and rub in the butter as for scones. Add sufficient water and lemon juice to form a stiff dough. Knead into a ball and refrigerate. Roll out thinly and line a 30cm pie dish. Bake at 210°C (400°F) for 10 minutes or until crust is cooked. Allow to cool and fill.

Filling

500g fresh ricotta cheese
½ cup evaporated milk
2 bananas, mashed
4 passionfruit
3 tablespoons lemon juice
extra passionfruit, strawberries or kiwi fruit

Combine ricotta and milk and beat until smooth. Fold in fruit and lemon juice. Pour into the baked pie crust and refrigerate until set. Decorate with extra passionfruit, slices of strawberry or kiwi fruit.

Serves 4-6

CHEESE CAKE

Crust

1 tablespoon butter
1 egg
1 cup wholemeal self raising flour

Lightly grease a 20cm spring form baking tin. Melt butter in a saucepan. Remove from heat and add well beaten egg. Add flour and mix well. Line base of prepared tin with pastry dough.

Filling

500g fresh ricotta or cottage cheese
1 cup plain yoghurt
3 eggs, separated
1 teaspoon vanilla

1 tablespoon lemon juice
grated rind 1 lemon
¼ cup honey
¼ cup brown rice flour

Place all filling ingredients except egg whites into a bowl and blend until smooth. Use a food processor if available. Beat egg whites until stiff and fold into cheese mixture. Pour filling into crust and bake at 180°C (350°F) until the centre is firm (approximately 45 minutes). Remove cake from oven and run a knife around the edge of the tin to loosen sides. Allow to cool before removing from tin. Top with yoghurt or Home Made Sour Cream (p. 100) and decorate with fresh berries or other fruit.

Serves 4-6

WAFFLES

1 cup soy beans
1¼ cups oatmeal
1½ cups water
1 tablespoon oil

Place the soy beans in a dish, add sufficient water to cover and leave to soak overnight. Drain and combine with other ingredients in a blender or food processor until light and airy. Pour into pre-heated waffle iron and cook for 15 minutes on medium heat. Do not open waffle iron for 15 minutes. Serve with fresh or stewed fruit.

Makes 8

BANANA PANCAKES

1 cup wholemeal plain flour
1 banana, mashed
½ teaspoon lemon juice
1 teaspoon lemon rind, grated
skim milk

Combine all ingredients, stirring in the milk to obtain a smooth paste. Drop spoonfuls onto a hot pan or skillet. Turn to cook the other side when bubbles appear on the top.

Makes 4-6 pancakes

YOGHURT PARFAIT

500g natural yoghurt
4 passionfruit
2 bananas
1 punnet strawberries or raspberries

Combine all ingredients. Spoon into tall glasses and decorate with extra chopped fruit or some finely chopped nuts. Any combination of fresh fruits can be used although the passion-fruit pulp is particularly delicious.

Serves 4

Beverages

When beginning the anti-Candida diet it is essential that alcohol is avoided. A small amount of distilled spirits with a low kilojoule mixer is allowed in Stage 2 of the diet but wine and beer must be eliminated until you reach the testing stage. However, refreshing, non-alcoholic drinks can be made easily at home and enjoyed as part of the diet.

FRUIT PUNCH

2 cups low kilojoule dry ginger ale
4 cups low kilojoule lemonade
juice of 2 lemons
4 passionfruit
1 tablespoon mint, finely chopped
1 lemon, thinly sliced
6 drops Angostura Bitters

Combine the ingredients in a large bowl or jug just before serving.

SUMMER FIZZ ◇Ⓛ

½ cup lemon or orange juice, freshly squeezed
1 cup mineral water

Combine ingredients and pour over ice in serving glasses.

FRUITY DELIGHT ◇

1½ cups Home Made Buttermilk (p. 117)
1½ cups orange juice, freshly squeezed

Combine ingredients in a blender or food processor and blend until smooth. Serve chilled.

STRAWBERRY DELIGHT ◇

1 cup Home Made Buttermilk (p. 117)
1 cup strawberries

Combine ingredients in a blender or food processor and blend until smooth. Serve chilled.

WATERMELON SURPRISE ◇

3 cups watermelon balls or cubes
2 cups ice cubes
1 sprig mint

Combine all ingredients in a blender or food processor and blend until light and frothy.

LIZZIE'S SPECIAL ◇

2 cups soda or mineral water
juice of 1 lime or lemon

2 drops Angostura Bitters
ice blocks
mint

Combine all ingredients except the mint and mix thoroughly.
Use the mint as a garnish.

ICED TEA ◊

1 pot weak tea, strained and cooled
ice cubes
lemon slices

Pour tea into a glass jug. Add ice cubes and lemon slices.
Chill well.

Some Home Made Everyday Foods

HOME MADE YOGHURT

1 litre skim milk
4 tablespoons skim milk powder
2 tablespoons commercially made natural yoghurt

Combine milk and milk powder in a saucepan and stir until combined. Gently heat milk to boiling point and then allow to cool to room temperature. Add a little of the milk to the yoghurt and blend until smooth. Combine with the rest of the milk, stirring well. Pour into a sterilised vacuum flask and allow to stand for 4-6 hours. The mixture should set to a firm yoghurt. Store in the refrigerator.

Variation Combine 1½ cups skim milk powder with 600ml hot water. Blend, as above, with 3 cups of commercially made yoghurt. Allow to set and store as above.

RICOTTA

4½ litres skim milk
3 tablespoons lemon juice, freshly squeezed

Gently heat milk to boiling point and then remove from heat immediately. Add lemon juice and allow to stand for 20 minutes. Strain to separate curds from the whey. Press curds firmly to remove as much liquid as possible. Remove to a covered container and store in the refrigerator.

Makes 2 cups

COTTAGE CHEESE

4 cups skim milk
1 plain junket tablet
1 tablespoon water

Dissolve crushed junket tablet in water in a large bowl. Heat milk until lukewarm and pour over dissolved junket tablet. Allow to stand in a warm place until set. When set, chop curds roughly and then pour cheese through a strainer which has been lined with muslin. When most of the liquid has been removed, gather the corners of the muslin and tie firmly, rather like a pudding. Hang in a cool place to allow whey to completely drain. This will take some hours and can be left overnight. Remove cheese from the cloth, place in an airtight container and store in the refrigerator. This will keep for up to 4 days.

Makes 1½ cups

HOME MADE BUTTERMILK

1 cup skim milk
2 teaspoons lemon juice

Combine ingredients and store in refrigerator.

Makes 1 cup

ALMOND CASHEW BUTTER

½ cup almonds
½ cup cashews
1 tablespoon vegetable oil
salt

Combine nuts and grind to a fine powder. Gradually add oil until a firm paste forms. Add salt if desired. Store in the refrigerator. This makes an excellent substitute for peanut butter.

Makes 1 cup

STRAWBERRY JAM

250g fresh strawberries
4 Granny Smith apples, peeled and cored
2 cups orange juice, freshly squeezed
1 teaspoon cinnamon
rind of 1 orange

Grate the apple and combine with the washed strawberries in a saucepan. Add the remaining ingredients and slowly bring to the boil. Simmer for 40 minutes or until thick, stirring occasionally. Pour into sterilised jars, cool and seal.
    Refrigerate after opening.

Makes 4 cups

STRAWBERRY TOPPING

1 cup ricotta cheese
½ cup natural yoghurt
1 cup strawberries, chopped

Mix cheese and yoghurt until smooth. Stir in the strawberries and serve with pancakes.

Makes 2½ cups

MUESLI   1 Serve = Ⓜ

Make fresh muesli every few days.

½ cup rolled oats
½ cup puffed rice
½ cup wholewheat flakes
2 teaspoons coconut, grated
2 tablespoons nuts, chopped

Serve with fresh fruit and either milk or yoghurt.

Makes 1¾ cups

CHAPTER 7

Vitamin and Mineral Supplements

A well balanced diet from a wide variety of food sources will usually provide an adequate supply of vitamins and minerals. However, if your diet is restricted by food allergies, your nutrient absorbtion disturbed because your gut is inflamed by Candida infestation, or your chemical load is heavier than normal, some nutrients may not be available to you and your vitamin and mineral requirements may be greater than normal. The severity of your allergic reaction may be lessened, and your recovery accelerated, by supplementing your diet with commercially available vitamins and minerals.

Vitamins and minerals are chemical substances which are essential to the body's chemistry but which cannot be manufactured by the body and so must be obtained from food sources. They are the building blocks of important hormones and enzymes which keep the body functioning. The whole range of vitamins and minerals, essential amino acids and fatty acids, is required for the normal functioning of the body.

In chronic Candidiasis and other allergy conditions, some nutrients are more important than others because either absorption is altered or more is needed by the body to deal with Candida toxins. Yeasts have their own range of essential nutrients. They thus compete with their host for these and may induce a nutrient deficiency in the host. In nutritional supplementation, the basic elements of Candidiasis treatment are employed: suppression of yeast while resting and assisting the immune system; recuperation of the immune system by providing it with more than adequate amounts of nutrients.

Because Candida imbalance produces a tendency to food intolerance, it is important when choosing a nutritional supplement to ensure that the preparation is free of any potentially allergic materials such as yeast, sugar, artificial colours and flavours, and is not derived from foods to which you are allergic such as wheat, dairy foods, soy, sugar cane or corn.

Here is a list of the nutrients which have been found to be helpful in treating Candidiasis.

Vitamin A

Adequate vitamin A is essential for the maintenance of healthy skin and mucous membranes and to resist the invasion of those surfaces by Candida and other infectious organisms. It is a basic ingredient of any supplement aimed at regeneration of a competent immune system. While supplementation or dietary sources may provide adequate vitamin A, its conversion to the active form which can be utilised by the body is dependent upon adequate zinc which is commonly deficient in Candida patients and so must also be supplemented.

Vitamin A is fat soluble so is stored in the body in fatty tissues. Over-supplementation can lead to toxic quantities of vitamin A being stored in the body so it is wise to use it only under supervision.

B Group Vitamins

There are many members of the family of B group vitamins which all have a degree of dependence on each other at all levels of the body's chemistry. When taking a B group vitamin, it is therefore important to ensure that the formula is properly balanced. Some of the B group members are more important for Candida patients and these are listed below.

Thiamine (Vitamin B1)

Some of the toxins produced by Candida are potent consumers of vitamin B1 in the liver so supplementation with vitamin B1 may help to reduce the ravages of these toxins.

Riboflavine (Vitamin B2)

Many of the unpleasant symptoms of Candidiasis are indicative of deficiency of vitamin B6 which depends for its activity upon the availability of sufficient riboflavine.

Pantothenic Acid (Vitamin B5)

Pantothenic acid deficiency severely inhibits antibody production, especially if there is a concurrent B6 deficiency, but this can be rectified by supplementation.

Pyridoxine (Vitamin B6)

Vitamin B6 has been identified as an important basic raw material for the establishment of a competent immune system. It has further been established that Candida toxins are great consumers of vitamin B6.

Vitamin B6 is an extremely important chemical in the body's basic chemistry. It is essential for the metabolism of fat and carbohydrate and for the maintenance of a proper level of blood glucose for the provision of energy. Red blood cells depend on vitamin B6 for their development and normal functioning. It is also the basis of the natural chemicals in the brain which prevent depression. Vitamin B6 is active in several different forms and these depend on the availability of zinc, magnesium and riboflavine for their conversion from one form to another.

Folic Acid

Folic acid is another of the B group vitamins without which immune function is impaired.

Vitamin C

Ascorbic acid (vitamin C) is one of the anti-oxidant vitamins (along with vitamin E and selenium) which is important as a de-toxifying agent in the removal of harmful allergic food substances, yeast metabolites and toxic chemicals. Vitamin C tidies up each cell's chemistry after the ravages of an invading harmful chemical. It is also important for the proper absorption of many minerals from the diet — especially zinc and iron. It is an essential part of any supplementation program aimed at reducing the load on the immune system.

Vitamin C, being water soluble, cannot be stored by the body so must be taken in divided doses throughout the day.

Vitamin E

The function of vitamin E in the body is similar to that of vitamin C and works together with vitamin C and selenium. Vitamin E is fat soluble so can be stored in the body and should not be taken in large doses unless supervised.

Zinc

One of the most important minerals for maintaining healthy skin and mucous membranes and for wound healing and resistance to infection is zinc. A deficiency leads to a breakdown of all facets of the immune system.

In Candida patients, it has been established that zinc deficiency is a common problem leading to a low immune system status, interference with essential fatty acid metabolism and with vitamin B6 metabolism leading to problems with red blood cell function and supply of energy requirements at a cellular level.

Supplementation with zinc will restore immune function and helps to overcome sugar craving.

Magnesium

Magnesium metabolism is closely allied with vitamin B6 metabolism so is extremely important for overcoming Candidiasis.

Iron

Maintenance of a competent immune system requires adequate iron in the body. A good diet would normally contain sufficient iron but its absorption may be compromised by an inflamed gut or lack of sufficient vitamin C.

Essential Amino Acids

Amino acids are the basic building blocks of protein in the body and are essential for the construction and repair of protein tissues including muscle and skin and as a substrate for most of the chemical reactions which occur within the body. These basic building blocks are obtained by digestion of protein in the diet. However, if protein digestion is incomplete or Candida in the gut competes for what is available, deficiencies of some amino acids will result.

The toxins of Candida interfere with the normal metabolism of amino acids resulting in their destruction, so a more than adequate supply is needed when Candida infection or infestation is present. The supply of sufficient amino acids can be enhanced by taking extra protein digesting enzymes or by directly supplementing with amino acids.

Essential Fatty Acids

The fats and oils which we consume consist wholly of fatty acids, most of which are nutritionally useless, while two are essential for normal functioning of the body's chemistry and for production of cell walls. Research has established that Candida patients have a tendency to have low levels of the essential fatty acids, alpha-linolenic acid and eicosapentanoic acid. These fatty acids are important in the production of prostaglandins (which suppress inflammatory reactions to toxins) and leukotrienes (which cause inflammatory reactions to toxins) where a predominance of the essential fatty acids tends to produce more prostaglandins and less leukotrienes.

Supplementation with linolenic acid from evening primrose oil or linseed oil and eicosapentanoic acid from cold water fish oils can enhance this effect.

Garlic

Garlic has been found to be actively anti-fungal in its effect and many people have found it helpful in overcoming Candida imbalance.

Lactobacillus Acidophilus

Lactobacillus acidophilus is the bacteria which is the culture medium used in the manufacture of some yoghurts and is also the bacteria which lives in competition with Candida in the gut. Its re-colonisation of the gut can be enhanced by taking extra yoghurt (sugar free) or by taking supplements of tablets of live cells of *Lactobacillus acidophilus*.

Supplementation of the diet with vitamins and minerals should enhance the recovery process when combatting Candida but is in no way a substitute for the diet described in this book.

Because of the possible toxicity of some vitamins and minerals when taken in excess, and because of the danger of a reaction to a non-active ingredient in commercial supplements, it is advisable to seek the advice of a health professional before adopting a course of supplementation.

CHAPTER 8

Exercise, Attitude and Your Environment

Research has shown the importance of exercise and relaxation. There is little to be gained sitting around, feeling miserable and sorry for yourself. Those who are physically fit and take a positive and responsible attitude to their own health reap the rewards.

Regular exercise is an important first step towards physical fitness. This can be enjoying your favourite sport, using an exercise bike or going for a daily walk. If you can manage a thirty minute walk at least five days a week the benefit will be enormous.

Start at your own pace and walk for fifteen minutes in one direction and then for fifteen minutes back again. You'll find that in a couple of weeks the distance you cover in thirty minutes will be much further than when you started. You may prefer to build yourself up to thirty minutes walking. Commence with ten minutes and keep extending the time every couple of days. You'll be pleased and possibly surprised with what you can achieve! It is important to walk without stopping to chat, or to look in shop windows or at neighbours' gardens.

Be happy and positive. If you are out somewhere and you cannot avoid eating some food which you have eliminated, don't despair. It will delay the time it takes to balance your yeasts and bacteria but all is not lost.

Your Environment

Now you have adjusted your diet and you are exercising happily, it is vital that you look at your environment and as far as possible avoid contact with mould. Often, it is not enough to merely remove yeast and mould products from the diet, it may be necessary to reduce the exposure to mould spores from the atmosphere. When a mould cell matures, it releases millions of tiny spores into the atmosphere, relying on wind and air currents to distribute the spores far and wide. The spores are inhaled along with air and are trapped by the normal air cleaning mechanisms on the mucous membranes of the nasal and chest airways. The spores can immediately initiate a local allergic reaction such as an attack of asthma, or may be carried along with the mucus to the throat and then swallowed. Mould metabolites released by decaying mould spores in the gut can be absorbed into the bloodstream and carried to the brain or other organs where they may cause a toxic reaction.

The environmental conditions which encourage mould growth are dampness and darkness, so attempts to control mould growth are aimed at establishing more light and dryer conditions.

Some old houses have a problem with rising damp. Is your house one of these? Is there a persistent mildew stain on the walls in one or more rooms? Is your house on the south side of the hill getting little sunlight. Seek advice on how to solve these problems and avoid sleeping in rooms which are damp or have any signs of mould in them.

Here are some other common sources of mould and ways of dealing with the problem.

Bathrooms often contain mould especially those which are poorly lit and poorly ventilated, particularly in the bath or shower area or in cupboards. Tile grouting, shower curtains, sliding shower screen tracks, damp and soiled towels and clothing are also sites which encourage mould growth.

Kitchens which have inadequate ventilation are a source of environmental mould contamination especially in under-sink cupboards, in refrigerator door seals and in the water evaporating tray under self-defrosting refrigerators. Check scored or worn wooden chopping boards. These should all be cleaned and aired frequently.

Bedrooms contain bedding which can become damp from perspiration which may not dry out in poorly ventilated rooms. This encourages mould growth. Regular laundering and airing of bedding will minimise this risk.

Cupboards and store rooms can be a source of mould, where soiled or old clothing, shoes, leather goods, newspapers, books etc. are stored. Clothes which are damp or have been worn and put away without laundering will quickly become mouldy while laundered clothing will keep well in a cupboard.

Damp under-house areas, cellars or sheds (especially those with an earth floor) have a high mould level and should be avoided.

Carpeting collects dust and mould in the pile which is not removed by normal vacuuming techniques. Scatter rugs can similarly become soiled unless laundered frequently.

Old upholstered or overstuffed furniture or bedding contains mould which cannot easily be removed by cleaning. Replace it if possible.

Indoor plants have soil and moisture in the pot along with decaying organic matter which encourages mould growth. Place them in well ventilated positions or remove them altogether.

Houses located in heavily timbered areas generally suffer from retained moisture which is not cleared because of shade and poor air circulation.

Decaying vegetable matter such as leaves and lawn clippings are very mouldy and mowing or raking will disturb millions of spores. Try to avoid these activities.

Fruits or vegetables stored in cupboards, pantry or sheds will quickly established moulds, especially root vegetables such as carrots and potatoes.

It may not be possible to remove or clean up all sources of mould exposure, but any improvement in the environment will certainly reduce the overall allergenic load and hopefully lead to an improvement and reduction of symptoms.

Index